CLARK'S POCKET HANDBOOK FOR

RADIOGRAPHERS

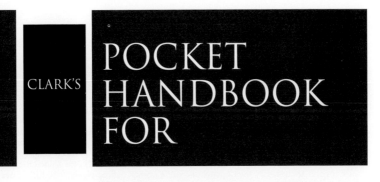

CLARK'S POCKET HANDBOOK FOR

RADIOGRAPHERS

Charles Sloane MSC DCR DRI Cert CI
Principal Lecturer and Radiography Course Leader,
University of Cumbria, Lancaster, UK

Ken Holmes MSC TDCR DRI Cert CI
Senior Lecturer, School of Medical Imaging Sciences,
University of Cumbria, Lancaster, UK

Craig Anderson MSC BSC
Clinical Tutor, X-ray Department,
Furness General Hospital, Cumbria, UK

A Stewart Whitley FCR TDCR HDCR FETC
Radiology Advisor, UK Radiology Advisory Services Ltd,
Preston, UK

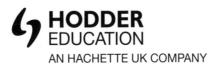

HODDER
EDUCATION
AN HACHETTE UK COMPANY

First published in Great Britain in 2010 by
Hodder Arnold, an imprint of Hodder Education, an Hachette UK company,
338 Euston Road, London NW1 3BH

http://www.hodderarnold.com

Hachette Livre UK's policy is to use papers that are natural, renewable and recyclable products
and made from wood grown in sustainable forests. The logging and manufacturing processes are
expected to conform to the environmental regulations of the country of origin.

Whilst the advice and information in this book are believed to be true and accurate at the date
of going to press, neither the authors nor the publisher can accept any legal responsibility or
liability for any errors or omissions that may be made. In particular, (but without limiting the
generality of the preceding disclaimer) every effort has been made to check drug dosages;
however it is still possible that errors have been missed. Furthermore, dosage schedules are
constantly being revised and new side-effects recognized. For these reasons the reader is
strongly urged to consult the drug companies' printed instructions before administering any
of the drugs recommended in this book.

British Library Cataloguing in Publication Data
A catalogue record for this book is available from the British Library

Library of Congress Cataloging-in-Publication Data
A catalog record for this book is available from the Library of Congress

ISBN-13 978-0-340-9 3993-2

1 2 3 4 5 6 7 8 9 10

Commissioning Editor:	Naomi Wilkinson
Project Editor:	Jane Tod
Production Controller:	Rachel Manguel
Cover Design:	Helen Townson
Indexer:	Lisa Footit

Typeset in 9.5/12 pt Berling Roman by MPS LIMITED, A Macmillan Company.
Printed and bound in Spain

What do you think about this book? Or any other Hodder Arnold title?
Please visit our website: www.hodderarnold.com

CONTENTS

Section 3 Useful Information for Radiographic Practice

PREFACE

This text is an accompaniment to the twelfth edition of *Clark's Positioning in Radiography*, a comprehensive bench-top guide to radiographic technique and positioning. The authors considered that it is important for radiographers and students to have access to an additional text available in a 'pocket' format which is easily transportable and convenient to use during everyday radiographic practice.

While it has been impossible to include all the radiographic projections from the twelfth edition due to size restrictions, the authors have included what they consider to be the most commonly used projections. Readers are advised to consult the twelfth edition of *Clark's Positioning in Radiography* if they seek guidance in undertaking any projections that have not been included within this book.

The authors have also included a range of additional information which is new to this text. This includes a protocol for evaluating images (the '10-point plan') and a range of general advice for undertaking procedures in a professional and efficient manner. The book also includes basic information in relation to some non-imaging diagnostic tests, common medical terminology and abbreviations. This is designed to help readers gain a better understanding of the diagnostic requirements and role of particular imaging procedures from the information presented in X-ray requests.

The various projections described in this book have been produced mainly from the twelfth edition of *Clark's Positioning in Radiography*. There have been some advances in technology which have changed the use of imaging equipment and terminology. This has been updated in the text of this edition but some of the images of radiographic positioning may not always reflect this. The main changes are outlined below.

The term 'focus film distance (FFD)' is now inappropriate due to the replacement of film technology with digital image acquisition technology. The term 'film' or 'film cassette' has been replaced with 'image receptor' or 'receptor'. The term 'focus film distance (FFD)' has been replaced with 'focus receptor distance (FRD)'. Unless otherwise stated the standard FRD for all examinations described is 110 cm.

When using film-based technology it was common practice to undertake two or more extremity examinations on one film/cassette, which was split into sections by the radiographer. If the radiographer is using computed radiography (CR) technology to acquire images, the advice of manufacturers is to undertake one image at a time in the middle of the CR cassette. Failure to do this may result in failure of the image-processing software to correctly identify the region of interest and the production of a sub-optimal image.

ACKNOWLEDGEMENTS

The authors would like to acknowledge the work of all the authors and the models who posed for the photographs of the twelfth edition of *Clark's Positioning in Radiography*, the book inspired by the original work and dedication of Kitty Clark and subsequent authors whose objective was to produce a meaningful and descriptive text for a new generation of radiographers. Special mention must also be given to Graham Hoadley, Consultant Radiologist, Blackpool Victoria Hospital, and Andrew Shaw, Clinical Scientist, Diagnostic Radiology and Radiation Protection Group, Christie Hospital, Manchester.

SECTION 1

KEY ASPECTS OF RADIOGRAPHIC PRACTICE

ANATOMICAL TERMINOLOGY

The human body is a complicated structure. Errors in radiographic positioning or diagnosis can easily occur unless practitioners have a common set of rules that are used to describe the body and its movements. All the basic terminology descriptions below refer to the patient in the standard reference position, known as the anatomical position (see opposite).

Patient Aspect

- Anterior aspect is that seen when viewing the patient from the front.
- Posterior (dorsal) aspect is that seen when viewing the patient from the back.
- Lateral aspect refers to any view of the patient from the side. The side of the head would therefore be the lateral aspect of the cranium.
- Medial aspect refers to the side of a body part closest to the midline, e.g. the inner side of a limb is the medial aspect of that limb.

Planes of the Body

Three planes of the body are used extensively for descriptions of positioning both in plain X-ray imaging as well as other cross-sectional imaging techniques. The planes described are mutually at right-angles to each other.

- Median sagittal plane (MSP) divides the body into right and left halves. Any plane parallel to this, but dividing the body into unequal right and left portions, is simply known as a sagittal plane or parasagittal plane.
- Coronal plane divides the body into an anterior part and a posterior part.
- Transverse or axial plane divides the body into a superior part and an inferior part.

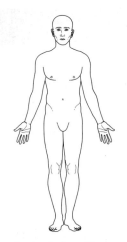

Anatomical position

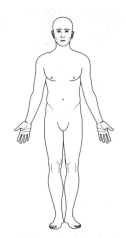

Anterior aspect of body

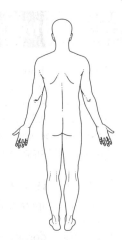

Posterior aspect of body

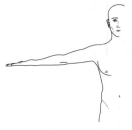

Medial aspect of arm

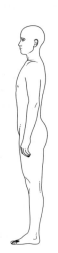

Lateral aspect of body

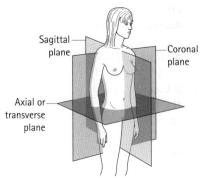

Sagittal plane

Coronal plane

Axial or transverse plane

Body planes

Lines and Landmarks Used in Radiography of the Skull

Landmarks

- Outer canthus of the eye: the point where the upper and lower eyelids meet laterally.
- Infra-orbital margin/point: the inferior rim of the orbit, with the point being located at its lowest point.
- Nasion: the articulation between the nasal and frontal bones.
- Glabella: a bony prominence found on the frontal bone immediately superior to the nasion.
- Vertex: the highest point of the skull in the median sagittal plane.
- External occipital protuberance (inion): a bony prominence found on the occipital bone, usually coincident with the median sagittal plane.
- External auditory meatus: the opening within the ear that leads into the external auditory canal.

Lines

- **Inter-orbital (interpupillary) line:** joins the centre of the two orbits or the centre of the two pupils when the eyes are looking straight forward.
- **Infra-orbital line:** joints the two infra-orbital points.
- **Anthropological baseline:** passes from the infra-orbital point to the upper border of the external auditory meatus (also known as the Frankfurter line).
- **Orbito-meatal baseline (radiographic baseline):** extends from the outer canthus of the eye to the centre of the external auditory meatus. This line is angled approximately 10 degrees to the anthropological baseline.

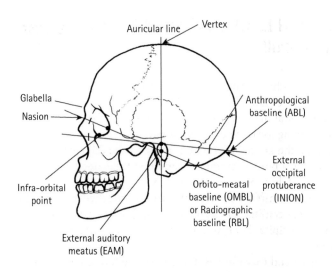

Auricular line — Vertex

Glabella

Nasion

Anthropological baseline (ABL)

External occipital protuberance (INION)

Infra-orbital point

Orbito-meatal baseline (OMBL) or Radiographic baseline (RBL)

External auditory meatus (EAM)

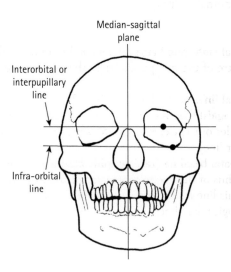

Median-sagittal plane

Interorbital or interpupillary line

Infra-orbital line

POSITIONING TERMINOLOGY

This section describes how the patient is positioned for the various radiographic projections described in this text.

Erect: the projection is taken with the patient sitting or standing:

- with the posterior aspect against the image receptor, or
- with the anterior aspect against the image receptor, or
- with the right or left side against the image receptor.

Decubitus: the patient is lying down. In the decubitus position the patient may be lying in any of the following positions:

- **supine (dorsal decubitus):** patient lying on their back.
- **prone (ventral decubitus):** lying face down.
- **lateral decubitus:** lying on the side: right lateral decubitus – lying on right side; left lateral decubitus – lying on left side.

Semi-recumbent: the patient is reclining, part way between supine and sitting erect.

All the positions may be more precisely described by reference to the planes of the body. For example, 'the patient is supine with the median sagittal plane at right-angles to the table top' or 'the patient is erect with the left side in contact with the image receptor and the coronal plane perpendicular to the image receptor'.

When describing positioning for upper limb projections the patient will often be 'seated by the table'. The photograph opposite (top left) shows the correct position to be used for upper limb radiography, with the coronal plane approximately perpendicular to the short axis of the tabletop. The legs will not be under the table, therefore avoiding exposure of the gonads to any primary radiation not attenuated by the image receptor or table.

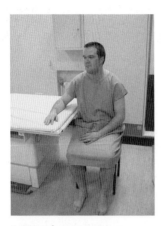

Position for extremity
radiography

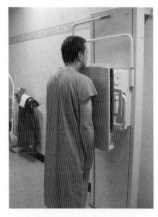

Erect, anterior aspect against
Bucky

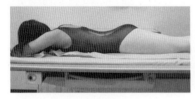

Prone

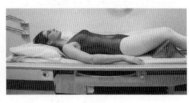

Supine

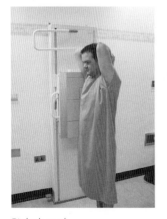

Right lateral

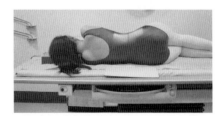

Left lateral decubitus

Terminology Used to Describe the Limb Position

Positioning for limb radiography may include:

- a description of the aspect of the limb in contact with the image receptor;
- direction of rotation of the limb in relation to the anatomical position, e.g. medial (internal) rotation toward the midline or lateral (external) rotation away from the midline;
- the final angle to the image receptor of a line joining two imaginary landmarks;
- movements and degree of movement of the various joints concerned.

Extension: when the angle of the joint increases.

Flexion: when the angle of the joint decreases.

Abduction: refers to a movement away from the midline.

Adduction: refers to a movement towards the midline.

Rotation: movement of the body part around its own axis, e.g. medial (internal) rotation towards the midline or lateral (external) rotation away from the midline.

Supination: a movement of the hand and forearm in which the palm is moved from facing anteriorly (as per anatomical position) to posteriorly.

Pronation: the reverse of supination. Other movement terms applied to specific body parts are described in the diagrams below.

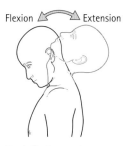

Neck flexion and extension

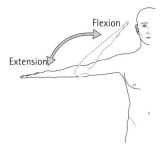

Elbow flexion and extension

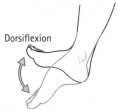

Dorsiflexion

Plantarflexion

Foot: dorsi and plantar flexion

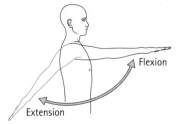

Flexion

Extension

Shoulder flexion and extension

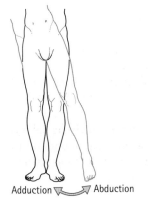

Adduction   Abduction

Hip adduction and abduction

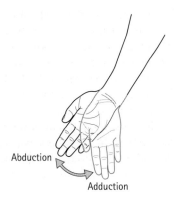

Abduction

Adduction

Wrist adduction and abduction

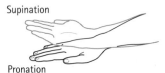

Supination

Pronation

Hand pronation and supination

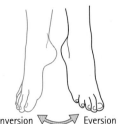

Inversion   Eversion

Foot inversion and eversion

PROJECTION TERMINOLOGY

A radiographic **projection** is described by the direction of the central ray relative to aspects and planes of the body.

Antero-posterior (AP)

The central ray is incident on the anterior aspect, passes along or parallel to the median sagittal plane and emerges from the posterior aspect of the body.

Postero-anterior (PA)

The central ray is incident on the posterior aspect, passes along or parallel to the median sagittal plane and emerges from the anterior aspect of the body.

Lateral

The central ray passes from one side of the body to the other along a coronal and transverse plane. The projection is called a right lateral if the central ray enters the body on the left side and passes through to the image receptor positioned on the right side. A left lateral is achieved if the central ray enters the body on the right side and passes through to the image receptor, which will be positioned parallel to the median sagittal plane on the left side of the body.

In the case of a limb the central ray is either incident on the lateral aspect and emerges from the medial aspect (latero-medial) or is incident on the medial aspect and emerges from the lateral aspect of the limb (medio-lateral). The terms 'latero-medial' and 'medio-lateral' are used where necessary to differentiate between the two projections.

Beam Angulation

Radiographic projections are often modified by directing the central ray at some angle to a transverse plane, i.e. either caudally (angled towards the feet) or cranially/cephalic angulation (angled towards the head). The projection is then described as, for example, a lateral 20-degree caudad or a lateral 15-degree cephalad.

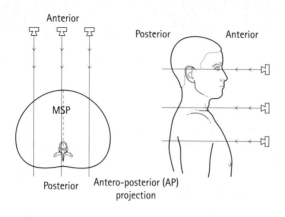

Antero-posterior (AP)
projection

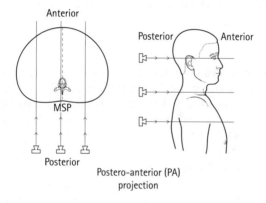

Postero-anterior (PA)
projection

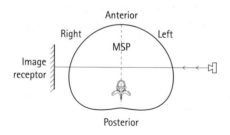

Right lateral projection

Oblique

The central ray passes through the body along a transverse plane at some angle between the median sagittal and coronal planes. For this projection the patient is usually positioned with the median sagittal plane at some angle between 0 and 90 degrees to the receptor with the central ray at right-angles to the receptor. If the patient is positioned with the median sagittal plane at right-angles to or parallel to the receptor the projection is obtained by directing the central ray at some angle to the median sagittal plane.

Anterior Oblique

The central ray enters the posterior aspect, passes along a transverse plane at some angle to the median sagittal plane and emerges from the anterior aspect. The projection is also described by the side of the torso closest to the cassette. In the diagram opposite the left side is closest to the cassette therefore the projection is a described as a left anterior oblique.

Posterior Oblique

The central ray enters the anterior aspect, passes along a transverse plane at some angle to the median sagittal plane and emerges from the posterior aspect. Again the projection is described by the side of the torso closest to the receptor. The diagram opposite shows a left posterior oblique.

Oblique Using Beam Angulation

When the median sagittal plane is at right-angles to the receptor, right and left anterior or posterior oblique projections may be obtained by angling the central ray to the median sagittal plane. NB This cannot be done if using a grid unless the grid lines are parallel to the central ray.

Lateral Oblique

The central ray enters one lateral aspect, passes along a transverse plane at an angle to the coronal plane and emerges from the opposite lateral aspect.

With the coronal plane at right-angles to the receptor, lateral oblique projections can also be obtained by angling the central ray to the coronal plane. NB This cannot be done if using a grid unless the grid lines are parallel to the central ray.

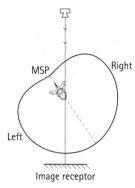

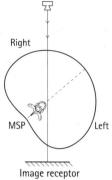

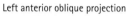

Image receptor

Left anterior oblique projection

Image receptor

Left posterior oblique projection

NB All diagrams are viewed as if looking upwards from the feet.

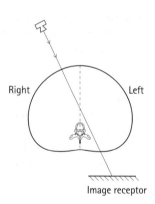

Image receptor

Left posterior oblique
obtained using an angled
beam

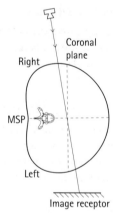

Image receptor

Left lateral oblique
projection

GENERAL CONSIDERATIONS FOR THE CONDUCT OF RADIOGRAPHIC EXAMINATIONS

Patient Considerations

- Always introduce yourself to the patient and state your profession.
- Explain the procedure and the patient's role.
- Rehearse any breathing manoeuvres (or similar) if the patient has a limited ability to cooperate.
- Check if the patient has complied with any preparation instructions (e.g. have they removed relevant clothing or jewellery?).
- Ask if the patient has any questions or concerns.
- After the examination inform the patient what they should do next and check they understand the advice given.

Procedural Considerations

- Always prepare the X-ray room for the procedure prior to the patient entering the room.
- Follow departmental protocols for the examination, e.g. the focus receptor distance (FRD), normally 110 cm unless otherwise stated.
- If using computed radiography:
  1 do not take multiple projections on one receptor/plate as this will confuse image processing algorithms;
  2 use the smallest receptor size consistent with size of the body part to maximize resolution.
- Always collimate to the area of interest as excessive field sizes reduce image quality and increase patient dose.
- It is best practice to apply anatomical side markers at the time of the examination and not to use electronic markers when post processing the image.

PATIENT IDENTITY AND CONSENT

Introduction

It is essential that the radiographer establishes a rapport with the patient and carers. The radiographer must first introduce him or herself and inform the patient/carer what to expect the during the examination. Then they must make sure the request form is for the patient being examined and the clinical details and history are accurate. The patient/carer's consent must be requested before the examination starts.

Request Form

The radiographer checks the request form to ensure the examination is justified according to:

- ionizing radiation regulations
- department protocols, making sure all the required details are on the form, i.e. patient demographics, examination requested, authorized signature for the examination and rationale for the examination.

An explanation of the examination is provided.

Patient Identity and Consent

- The identity is established using the departmental protocol, which normally asks the patient to state their full name, address and date of birth. These are then cross-referenced with the request form. The examination must not proceed unless the radiographer is sure of the identity of the patient
- The procedure is explained to the patient in easy to understand terms avoiding medical jargon.

The patient is asked:

- if they have undertaken any required preparation for the examination;
- if they understand the nature of the examination and if they have any questions prior to proceeding;
- for verbal permission to proceed with the examination;

- for written consent if an examination incurs a higher risk, e.g. angiography.

To be able to give consent (adult or child) the patient should meet the following criteria:

- they should understand the risk versus benefit;
- they should understand the nature of the examination and why it is being performed;
- they should understand the consequences of not having the examination;
- they should be able to make and communicate an informed decision.

If these conditions are not fulfilled then other individuals may be able to give consent, e.g. parents, or in an emergency situation the examination may proceed if it is considered in the best interest of the patient (see hospital policy).

JUSTIFICATION OF EXAMINATION

Upon receipt of a request for an X-ray examination, the radiographer needs to carefully consider if the requested examination is appropriate to undertake. In other words – is the examination justified?

The radiographer should consider several questions when assessing any request for imaging:

- **Will the examination change the clinical management of the patient?**

  Although this can be a contentious area, the radiographer should consider if the requested examination will be of benefit to the patient and if the findings will affect the treatment or management of the patient.

- **Does the completed request comply with local protocol?**

  For example, is the request card completed in a legible manner? Are the patient demographics correct? Is the requested examination in line with the departmental protocol? Is the referrer identified and working within their referral protocol?

- **Are the details of previous operations or other relevant recent imaging included?**

  This may have a bearing on the projections taken or the validity of the requested examination.

- **What are the risks/benefits of the examination?**

  Even low X-ray doses can cause changes to cell DNA, leading to increased probability of cancer occurring in the years following the exposure. Although in many cases the probability of this occurring is low, the risk of this occurring should always be balanced against the benefits of the patient undergoing the examination. This is often acutely emphasized when seriously ill patients undergo frequent X-ray examinations and the need to carefully consider each request is very important. Consultation with radiological colleagues is often required if there is any doubt over the legitimacy of any request.

- **Does the request comply with government legislation?**

  Legislation varies between countries; however, the request should comply with national legislation where applicable. In the UK the underlying legislation is known as the Ionising Radiation (Medical

Exposure) Regulations (IR(ME)R) 2000. This legislation is designed to protect patients by keeping doses as low as reasonably practicable. (ALARP). The regulations set out responsibilities for those who refer patients for an examination (referrers); those who *justify* the exposure to take place (practitioners); and those who undertake the exposure (operators). Radiographers frequently act as practitioners and as such must be aware of the legislation along with the risks and benefits of the examination to be able to justify it.

■ **Is there an alternative imaging modality?**
The use of an alternative imaging modality that may provide more relevant information or the information required at a lower dose should be considered. The use of non-ionizing imaging modalities, such as ultrasound and magnetic resonance (MRI), should also be considered where appropriate.

RADIATION PROTECTION

The following is a list of general principles that can be followed to minimize dose to patients and staff at various stages of the radiological examination.

Patient

- Explain the procedure to the patient and the need to keep still.
- Make the patient comfortable.

Other Staff and Carers

- Only required staff in the X-ray room.
- If supporting the patient, use lead protection.

Radiographer

- Justify the request.
- X-ray the correct patient: check two forms of ID.
- X-ray the correct body part (check against body part on request card and patient history.
- Collimate to the area of interest.
- Careful technique (no repeated examinations).
- Use optimum exposure factors (dose reference levels are a legal requirement of practice).
- Optimum beam energy (kVp) used for examination and imaging system.
- Stand behind radiation barrier.
- Don't point the X-ray tube in the direction of the radiation barrier or doors (which must be closed).

Additional Considerations

- Prepare the room and set a preliminary exposure before inviting the patient into the X-ray room.
- Always explain what you are trying to achieve and what is expected of the patient.

- Equipment must have regular QA checks to ensure it is working at the optimum level.

If a patient is worried about the radiation dose they might receive you can use the following statements to put the risk into context.

- You have more chance of drowning in the bath in the next year than you have of getting cancer from a chest/extremity X-ray.
- An abdomen X-ray carries about the same risk of death as playing a game of football.
- A computed tomography (CT) head examination carries approximately the same risk of death that the average UK road user faces per year.

Table 1.1 Radiation dose quantities

Dose quantities	Unit	Definition
Absorbed dose	Gy	Energy absorbed in a known mass of tissue
Organ dose	mGy	Average dose to specific tissue
Effective dose	mSv	Overall dose weighted for sensitivity of different organs; indicates risk
Entrance surface dose	mGy	Dose measured at beam entrance surface; used to monitor doses and set DRLs for radiographs
Dose–area product	Gy per cm^2	Product of dose (in air) and beam area; used to monitor doses and set DRLs for examinations

DRL, dose reference level.

Table 2.2 Radiations risk for X-ray examinations to an average adult

Examination	Typical effective dose (mSv)	Risk*
Hand/foot	0.01	1 in a few million
Chest	0.02	1 in 1 000 000
Mammography	0.06	1 in 300 000
Abdomen	0.7	1 in 30 000
Lumbar spine	1.3	1 in 15 000
CT head	2	1 in 10 000
Barium enema	7.2	1 in 2800
CT body	9	1 in 2200

*Additional lifetime risk of fatal cancer.

CT, computed tomography.

PREGNANCY

Avoiding Exposure in Pregnancy

All imaging departments should have written procedures for managing the small but significant radiation risk to the fetus. Radiographers should refer to their departmental working procedures and apply them as part of their everyday working practice.

The chart opposite has been constructed using joint guidance from the UK National Radiation Protection Board, the College of Radiographers and the Royal College of Radiologists (1998). Most departmental procedures will follow a similar procedure although practices may vary between departments according to specific circumstances.

The procedure for pregnancy is usually applied to examinations that involve the primary beam exposing the pelvic area. Examinations of other areas can be undertaken as long as the radiographer ensures good beam collimation and employs the use of lead protection for the pelvis.

Evaluating and Minimizing the Radiation Risks in Pregnancy

If a decision is made to irradiate a woman who is pregnant it will be in conjunction with the referring clinician who will have decided that there are overriding clinical reasons for the examination to take place.

In such cases the relatively small radiation risk to the patient/fetus will be outweighed by the benefit of the diagnosis and subsequent treatment of potentially life-threatening or serious conditions. These could present a much greater risk to both parties if left undiagnosed.

To minimize the risks when examining pregnant women the radiographer should adopt the following strategies:

- use of the highest imaging speed system available, e.g. 800 speed;
- close collimation to area of interest;
- use of shielding (can the uterus be shielded without significant loss of diagnostic information?);
- use of the minimum number of exposures to establish a diagnosis;
- use of projections that give the lowest doses;
- consider the use of pregnancy tests if doubt exists.[†]

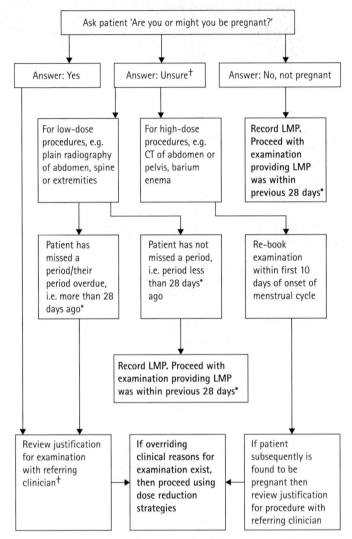

A typical 'pregnancy rule' for women of child-bearing age. *Some women have menstrual cycles of more or less than 28 days or have irregular cycles. CT, computed tomography; LMP, last menstrual period.

EVALUATING IMAGES: 'THE 10-POINT PLAN'

It is imperative that radiographic images are properly evaluated to ensure that they are fit for purpose, i.e. they must answer the diagnostic question posed by the clinician making the request. In order to do this effectively the person undertaking the evaluation must be aware of the radiographic appearances of potential pathologies and the relevant anatomy that needs to be demonstrated by a particular projection.

Points to Consider When Evaluating the Suitability of Radiographs

1 **Patient identification:** do the details on the image match those on the request card and those of the patient who was examined? Such details may include patient name and demographics, accession number, date of examination and the name of the hospital.

2 **Area of interest:** does the radiograph include all the relevant areas of anatomy? The anatomy that needs to be demonstrated may vary depending on the clinical indications for the examination.

3 **Markers and legends:** check that the correct anatomical side markers are clearly visible in the radiation field. Ensure the marker that has been used matches the body part on the radiograph and that this in turn matches the initial request from the clinician. Ensure the correct legends have been included if not stated in the examination protocol, e.g. prone/supine. It is poor practice not to include a marker within the radiation field when making an exposure.

4 **Correct projection:** has the patient been positioned correctly and does this positioning follow departmental protocols? Positioning that matches strict evaluation criteria may not always be required. It is important to consider the pathology in question and the clinical presentation of the patient. If debating whether a projection is acceptable always consider if the 'diagnostic question' has been answered.

5 **Correct image exposure:** the evaluation of the appropriateness of the exposure factors used for a radiograph will depend on the equipment used to obtain the image.

Conventional Film-based Imaging

- *Image density*: the degree of film blackening should allow relevant anatomy to be sufficiently demonstrated, thus allowing diagnosis.
- *Image contrast*: the range of useful densities produced on the radiographic image should correspond to the structures within the area of interest. Each anatomical area should be of sufficient density to allow relevant anatomical structures to be clearly visualized.

Digital Image Capture Systems

Given the wide exposure latitude of digital systems the primary task when evaluating the image is to assess for over- and underexposure. The imaging equipment will usually give a numerical indication of the exposure used, the detector dose indicator (DDI). The reading is compared with a range of exposure limits provided by the manufacturer to see if it is above or below recommended values.

Underexposure: images that are underexposed will show unacceptable levels of 'noise' or 'mottle' even though the computer screen brightness (image density) will be acceptable (see image, page 27).

Overexposure: image quality will actually improve as exposure increases due to lower levels of noise. Once a certain point is reached, further increases in exposure will result in reduced contrast. Eventually a point is reached when the image contrast becomes unacceptable (see image, page 27).

NB: There is considerable scope for exposing patients to unnecessarily high doses of radiation using digital imaging technologies. When evaluating images it is important to always use the lowest dose that gives an acceptable level of image noise and to compare doses used with national dose reference levels.

6 **Optimum resolution:** is the image sharp? Look at bone cortices and trabeculae to ensure movement or other factors have not caused an unacceptable degree of unsharpness.

7 **Collimation:** has any of the area of interest been missed due to over-zealous collimation? Check relevant soft tissues have been included. Also look for signs of collimation to evaluate the success of the collimation strategy you used. This can then be used for future reference when performing similar examinations.

8 **Artefacts:** are there any artefacts on the image? These may be from either the patient or the imaging process. Only repeat if the artefact is interfering with diagnosis.

9 **Need for repeat radiographs or further projections:** a judgement is made from evaluations 1–8. If one or more factors have reduced the diagnostic quality to a point where a diagnosis cannot be made the image should be repeated. Would any additional projections enhance the diagnostic potential of the examination? For example, radial head projections for an elbow radiograph. If a repeat is required it may be appropriate to image only the area where there was uncertainty in the initial image.

10 **Anatomical variations and pathological appearances:** note anything unusual such as normal variants or pathology that may influence your future actions (see point 9) or aid diagnosis. For example, if an old injury is seen it may be worth questioning the patient about their medical history. This could then be recorded to aid diagnosis.

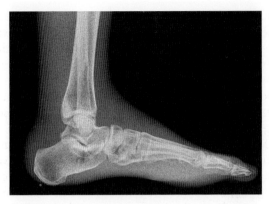

Underexposed digital radiograph

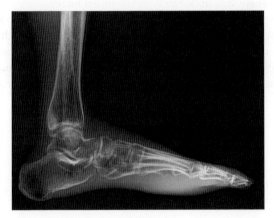

Overexposed digital radiograph

EXAMINATION TIMELINE

The following checklist summarizes the radiographer's role and the various stages that are followed during an imaging procedure.

1 Preparation
Procedure
- Review imaging request form
- Justification of the examination
- Check previous studies
- Review relevant departmental protocols
- Infection control considerations (e.g. MRSA)
- Consider specific radiation protection requirements

X-ray Room
- Room safe and tidy
- Optimization of exposure. X-ray generator set for correct procedure
- Tube positioned for procedure
- Prepare image receptors/cassettes
- Accessory equipment available

Patient
- Communicate effectively
- Introduce yourself and state your profession
- Correctly identify patient
- Check pregnancy status
- Explain procedure and gain consent
- Prepare patient if necessary, e.g. request they change into a gown

2 Examination
Patient Care
- Wash/clean your hands in sight of the patient
- Communicate effectively
- Be friendly and sympathetic

- Give clear instructions
- Explain what you are doing
- Explain why you are doing it
- Invite and answer any questions

Radiographic Procedure

- X-ray correct patient
- Follow department protocols
- Use a precise technique
- Be quick, safe and efficient
- Get it right first time
- Wash/clean hands following the procedure

Radiation Protection

- Correct protocol
- Only essential people in the room
- Use optimal exposure
- Collimate to area of interest
- Apply lead protection if appropriate

3 Aftercare

Assessment of Image Quality (10-Point Plan)

1 Patient identification
2 Area of interest
3 Markers and legends included in image
4 Correct projection
5 Correct exposure
6 Optimum resolution
7 Collimation to area of interest
8 Artefacts
9 Need for repeat radiographs or further projections
10 Anatomical variations and pathological appearances

Patient

- Communicate effectively
- Explain what they need to do next

- Invite and answer any questions
- Arrange transport if necessary

Case Review

- Request card completed
- Red dot or consider contacting referrer if major pathology
- Check images are archived in the correct folder
- Update radiology information system (RIS) and close examination

GUIDELINES FOR THE ASSESSMENT OF TRAUMA

Background

Radiographers are well placed to offer opinions on trauma plain radiographic images and can assist the referring clinician with identification of fractures, dislocations and associated 'signs', such as fluid levels. In the UK the practice of 'red-dotting' is well established and involves the radiographer placing a red dot or similar marker on the image to indicate the presence of an abnormality.

Developments in the Role of the Radiographer

In the UK, the basic system of placing a red dot has developed into a three-tier system of radiographer opinion:

1 **Red dot** – a basic system of flagging a possible abnormality, such as a fracture.
2 **Comment system** – the radiographer attaches a simple comment to the image to explain their concern.
3 **Clinical report** – trained radiographers produce a detailed report, usually some time after the examination, that is sent to the referring clinician.

Most radiographers, especially newly qualified practitioners will be working to develop their skills on the 'red-dot' and 'commenting' systems.

Suggestions for Successful Image Interpretation

1 **Gain an oral clinical history** – Obtaining a clinical history from the patient can be especially helpful for the radiographer to produce the correct projections required to demonstrate the injury and a greater understanding of the area to check for injury. Modern Picture Archiving and Communication Systems (PACS) also allow the radiographer to convey any relevant clinical history to the person providing the final radiological report.

2 **Produce high-quality radiographs** – poor images are especially difficult to interpret and the ability to exclude fractures with confidence is diminished.

3 **Use a logical system for checking** – many different approaches to evaluate radiographs are suggested in the radiology literature, such as looking at alignment, then bones, followed by cartilage, etc. Many useful lines and measurements are used to check for abnormalities, for example 'McGrigor's three lines' for evaluating the facial bones. Whichever system you use, try to apply it consistently and logically, which should reveal many subtle injuries.

4 **Utilize a system of pattern recognition** – carefully trace the cortical outlines of each bone, looking for any steps, breaks or discontinuities. Radiographers are used to seeing a large amount of 'normal' examinations and as such are well placed to use this knowledge to identify any changes in the normal 'pattern' of bones and joints. After checking the cortical margins, carefully assess the cancellous components of the bones, looking for discontinuities in the trabecular pattern which may indicate a fracture.

5 **Pay attention to 'hot-spots'** – where frequent bony injuries occur, such as the neck of the fifth metacarpal, the base of the fifth metatarsal, the dorsal aspect of the distal radius or the supracondylar region of the humerus in children. Frequently, the way the patient presents or reacts to positioning gives strong clues as to the position of the injury.

6 **Be aware of the indirect signs of a fracture** – for example, be able to identify and recognize the significance of an elbow joint effusion or a lipohaemarthrosis (fat/blood interface within the knee or shoulder joint), all of which can be associated with an underlying fracture.

7 **Look for the second fracture** – There is an old saying 'if you spot one fracture, look for another' and a common mistake is to identify a fracture but miss a second by not checking the entire image. Be aware of principles such as the 'bony ring rule', which states that if a fracture or dislocation is seen within a bony ring (e.g. pelvis), then a further injury should be sought as there are frequently two fractures.

THEATRE RADIOGRAPHY

Introduction

Theatre radiography plays a significant role in the delivery of surgical services. The radiographer may be required for emergency procedures or planned surgery in both trauma and non-trauma procedures.

Considerations for the Radiographer

Liaison

- The radiographer must contact the theatre sister upon arrival and maintain a close liaison with all people performing the operation, consequently working as part of the multidisciplinary team.
- The radiographer must be familiar with the layout and protocols associated with the theatre to which they are assigned, demonstrate a working knowledge of the duties of each person in the operating theatre, and ascertain the specific requirements of the surgeon who is operating.

Preparation

- Personal preparation is the first concern of the radiographer before entering an aseptic controlled area.
- The radiographer removes their uniform (and any jewellery), and replaces them with theatre wear. The hair is covered completely with a disposable hat. Theatre shoes or boots are worn, and a facemask is put on. In addition, a radiation-monitoring badge is pinned to theatre garments.
- Special attention is made to washing the hands using soap, ensuring that the hands are washed before and after each patient. If the skin has an abrasion, this should be covered with a waterproof dressing.
- Image receptor holders, stationary grids and other imaging devices should be cleaned and checked if required.
- Contrast media, if required, should also be supplied to the theatre staff.

Equipment

- A mobile X-ray unit or mobile image intensifier is selected, depending on the requirement of the radiographic procedure, i.e. a mobile X-ray unit may be used for plain chest radiography, while a mobile image intensifier may be used for the screening of orthopaedic procedures such as hip pinning.
- Before use, an image intensifier should be assembled and tested ahead of the procedure to ensure that it is functioning effectively prior to patient positioning.
- Exposure parameters are then optimized for the patient.

PACS Connectivity

In many theatre suites it is customary for the X-ray equipment to be housed within the suite and a PACS/Digital Imaging and Communications in Medicine (DICOM) link should be established to facilitate image capture and retrieval of previous examinations. Patients need to be entered on the PACS prior to the procedure commencing to allow the images to be stored in the correct files.

Radiation Protection

- Radiation protection is the responsibility of the radiographer operating the X-ray equipment. Therefore, the radiographer should ensure that radiation-monitoring badges, lead protective aprons and thyroid shields are worn by all staff wherever possible. Furthermore, as soon as the imaging equipment is switched on, a controlled area exists. Therefore, all doors that have access to the controlled area should display radiation warning signs.
- The inverse square law principle must be applied in the theatre environment. Therefore, staff must be standing at the maximum distance from the source of radiation, and outside the path of the primary beam during exposure.
- The radiation field should be collimated to the area of interest and no more than the size of the image receptor. Image receptor support devices should be used if required.
- The radiographer should aim to maximize the use of dose-saving facilities while using an image intensifier, e.g. pulsed exposures.

- Patient identification and pregnancy status must be confirmed with either the anaesthetist or an appropriate member of the theatre team before any radiation exposure.
- Records should be kept of patient details, exposure time and radiation dose when screening is employed.
- The radiographer must give clear instructions to staff before exposures are made regarding their role in reducing the risk of accidental exposure.

Sterile Procedures

- The radiographer should avoid the contamination of sterile areas. Ideally, equipment should be positioned before any sterile towels are placed in position, and care should be exercised not to touch sterile areas when positioning the image receptor or moving equipment during the operation.
- For the prevention of infection, the unit selected should be cleaned and dried after each patient. Where appropriate, protective plastic coverings can be used to reduce blood contamination during surgical procedures. When blood or other bodily fluids do come into contact with the imaging equipment, an appropriate cleaning solution, as advised by the local infection control officer, should be used.

SECTION 2
RADIOGRAPHIC PROJECTIONS

ABDOMEN – ANTERO-POSTERIOR SUPINE

Position of Patient and Image Receptor

- The patient lies supine on the imaging table, with the median sagittal plane at right-angles and coincident with the midline of the table.
- The pelvis is adjusted so that the anterior superior iliac spines are equidistant from the tabletop.
- The image receptor is placed longitudinally in the Bucky tray and positioned so that the symphysis pubis is included on the lower part of the image receptor, bearing in mind that the oblique rays will project the symphysis pubis downwards.
- The centre of the image receptor will be approximately at the level of a point located 1 cm below the line joining the iliac crests. This will ensure that the symphysis pubis is included on the image.

Direction and Centring of X-ray Beam

- The vertical central ray is directed to the centre of the imaging receptor.
- Using a short exposure time, the exposure is made on arrested respiration.

Essential Image Characteristics

- The area of interest must include from the diaphragm to symphysis pubis and the lateral properitoneal fat stripes.
- The bowel pattern should be demonstrated with minimal unsharpness.

Additional Considerations

- The 'pregnancy rule' should be observed unless it has been decided to ignore it in the case of an emergency.
- Gonad shielding can be used, but not when there is a possibility that important radiological signs may be hidden.

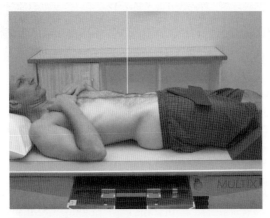

Positioning for supine abdomen

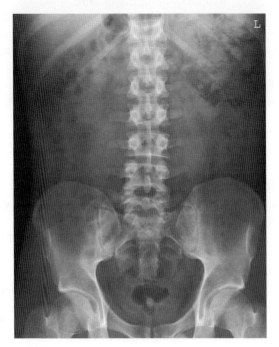

Radiograph of supine abdomen

ABDOMEN – PRONE

This projection is used to demonstrate the bowel in barium follow-through examinations. It may also be used in excretion urography and barium enema examinations.

Position of Patient and Image Receptor

- The patient lies prone with the legs extended and the head and arms resting on a pillow. The trunk is adjusted so that the median sagittal plane is at right-angles and the coronal plane is parallel to the image receptor.
- The pelvis is adjusted so that the posterior superior iliac spines are equidistant from the tabletop.
- The image receptor is placed longitudinally and positioned so that the symphysis pubis is included on the lower part of the image, bearing in mind that the oblique rays will project the symphysis pubis downwards.
- The centre of the image receptor will be approximately at the level of a point located 1 cm below the line joining the iliac crests. This will ensure that the symphysis pubis is included on the image.

Direction and Centring of X-ray Beam

The vertical central ray is directed to the centre of the image receptor.

Essential Image Characteristics

- The whole abdomen to include diaphragm to symphysis pubis and lateral flanks must be included.
- The bowel pattern should be demonstrated with minimal unsharpness.

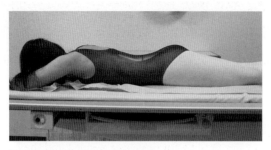

Positioning for prone abdomen

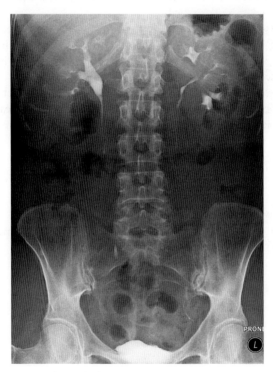

Prone radiograph (for intravenous urogram)

ABDOMEN – LEFT LATERAL DECUBITUS

This projection is used if the patient cannot be positioned erect or sitting to confirm the presence of sub-diaphragmatic gas suspected seen on the antero-posterior supine projection. It may also be used for confirming obstruction.

With the patient lying on the left side, free gas will rise, to be located between the lateral margin of the liver and the right lateral abdominal wall. To allow time for the gas to collect there, the patient should remain lying on the left side for 20 minutes before the exposure is made.

Position of Patient and Image Receptor
- The patient lies on the left side, with the elbows and arms flexed so that the hands can rest near the patient's head.
- The image receptor is positioned transversely against the posterior aspect of the trunk, with its upper border high enough to project above the right lateral abdominal and thoracic walls.
- A small region of the lung above the diaphragm should be included on the image.
- The patient's position is adjusted to bring the median sagittal plane at right-angles to the image receptor.

Direction and Centring of X-ray Beam
- The horizontal central ray is directed to the anterior aspect of the patient and centred to the centre of the image receptor.

Essential Image Characteristics
- The area of interest should include from the diaphragm to symphysis pubis and the lateral abdominal walls.
- The bowel pattern should be demonstrated with minimal unsharpness.

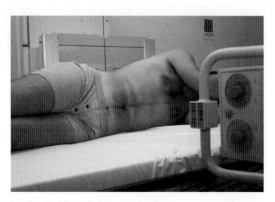

Positioning for left lateral decubitus

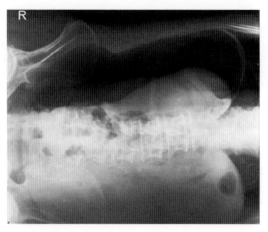

Radiograph of left lateral decubitus demonstrating free air (perforation)

ACROMIOCLAVICULAR JOINT

An antero-posterior projection of the joint in question is all that is normally required. In certain circumstances, subluxation of the joint may be confirmed with the patient holding a heavy weight.

Position of Patient and Image Receptor

- The patient stands facing the X-ray tube, with the arms relaxed to the side. The posterior aspect of the shoulder being examined is placed in contact with the image receptor, and the patient is then rotated approximately 15 degrees towards the side being examined to bring the acromioclavicular joint space at right-angles to the image receptor.
- The image receptor is positioned so that the acromion process is in the centre of the image receptor.

Direction and Centring of X-ray Beam

- The horizontal central ray is centred to the palpable lateral end of the clavicle at the acromioclavicular joint.
- To avoid superimposition of the joint on the spine of the scapula, the central ray can be angled 25 degrees cranially before centring to the joint.

Essential Image Characteristics

- The image should demonstrate the acromioclavicular joint and the clavicle projected above the acromion process.
- The exposure should demonstrate soft tissue around the articulation.

Notes

- The normal joint is variable (3–8 mm) in width. The normal difference between the sides should be less than 2–3 mm.[1]
- The inferior surfaces of the acromion and clavicle should normally be in a straight line.

[1]Manaster BJ (1997) *Handbook of Skeletal Radiology*, 2nd edn. St Louis: Mosby.

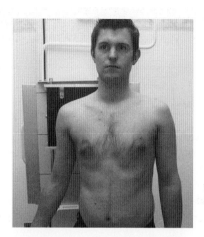

Positioning for acromioclavicular joint

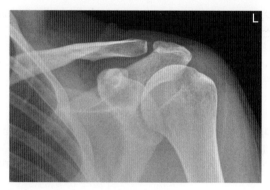

Radiograph of acromioclavicular joint

ANKLE – ANTERO-POSTERIOR/ MORTICE JOINT

Position of Patient and Image Receptor

- The patient is either supine or seated on the X-ray table with both legs extended.
- A pad may be placed under the knee for comfort.
- The affected ankle is supported in dorsiflexion by a firm 90-degree pad placed against the plantar aspect of the foot.
- The limb is rotated medially (approximately 20 degrees) until the medial and lateral malleoli are equidistant from the image receptor.
- The lower edge of the image receptor is positioned just below the plantar aspect of the heel.

Direction and Centring of X-ray Beam

- Centre midway between the malleoli with the vertical central ray at 90 degrees to an imaginary line joining the malleoli.

Essential Image Characteristics

- The lower third of the tibia and fibula should be included.
- A clear joint space between the tibia, fibula and talus should be demonstrated (commonly called the mortice view).

Additional Considerations

- Insufficient dorsiflexion = calcaneum superimposed on lateral malleolus.
- Insufficient internal rotation = overlapping of the tibiofibular joint.

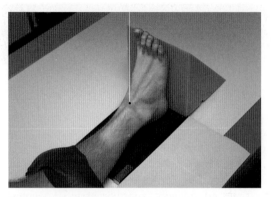

Positioning for antero-posterior ankle

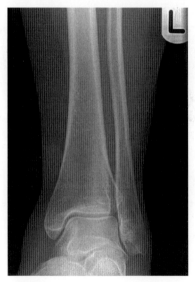

Example of antero-posterior ankle
radiograph

ANKLE – LATERAL

Position of Patient and Image Receptor

- With the ankle dorsiflexed, the patient turns onto the affected side until the malleoli are superimposed vertically and the tibia is parallel to the image receptor.
- A 15-degree pad is placed under the lateral border of the forefoot and a pad is placed under the knee for support. The lower edge of the image receptor is positioned just below the plantar aspect of the heel.

Direction and Centring of X-ray Beam

- Centre over the medial malleolus, with the central ray at right-angles to the axis of the tibia.

Essential Image Characteristics

- The lower third of the tibia and fibula should be included.
- The medial and lateral borders of the trochlear articular surface of the talus should be superimposed on the image.
- The base of fifth metatarsal should be included to exclude a fracture.

Additional Considerations

- Over- and under-rotation lead to non-superimposition of the talar trochlear surfaces.
- Over-rotation = fibula projected posterior to the tibia.
- Under-rotation = shaft of the fibula superimposed on the tibia.

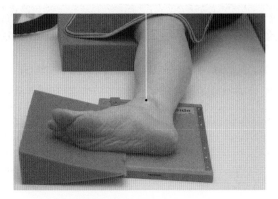

Positioning for lateral ankle

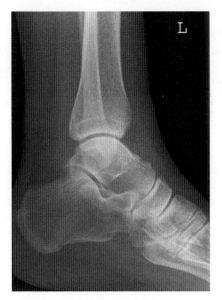

Example of lateral ankle radiograph

CALCANEUM – AXIAL

Position of Patient and Image Receptor

- The patient sits or lies supine on the X-ray table with both limbs extended.
- The affected leg is rotated medially until both malleoli are equidistant from the image receptor.
- The ankle is dorsiflexed. The position is maintained by using a bandage strapped around the forefoot and held in position by the patient.
- The image receptor is positioned with its lower edge just distal to the plantar aspect of the heel.

Direction and Centring of X-ray Beam

- Centre to the plantar aspect of the heel at the level of the base of the fifth metatarsal.
- The central ray is directed cranially at an angle of 40 degrees to the plantar aspect of the heel.

Essential Image Characteristics

- The subtalar joint should be visible on the axial projection.

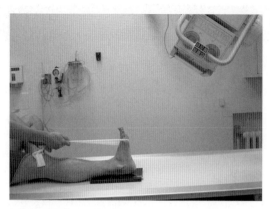

Positioning for axial calcaneum

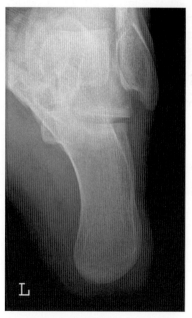

Example of axial calcaneum radiograph

CERVICAL SPINE –
ANTERO-POSTERIOR C3–C7

Position of Patient and Image Receptor

- The patient lies supine on the Bucky table or, if erect positioning is preferred, sits or stands with the posterior aspect of the head and shoulders against the vertical Bucky.
- The median sagittal plane is adjusted to be at right-angles to the image receptor and to coincide with the midline of the table or Bucky.
- The neck is extended (if the patient's condition will allow) so that the lower part of the jaw is cleared from the upper cervical vertebra.
- The image receptor/Bucky is positioned to coincide with the central ray. The Bucky will require some cranial displacement if the tube is angled.

Direction and Centring of X-ray Beam

- A 5- to 15-degree cranial angulation is employed, such that the inferior border of the symphysis menti is superimposed over the occipital bone.
- The beam is centred in the midline towards a point just below the prominence of the thyroid cartilage through the fifth cervical vertebra.

Essential Image Characteristics

- The image must demonstrate the third cervical vertebra down to the cervical-thoracic junction.
- Lateral collimation to soft tissue margins.
- The chin should be superimposed over the occipital bone.

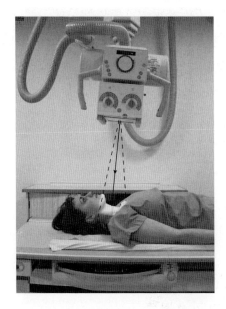

Positioning for
antero-posterior
cervical spine

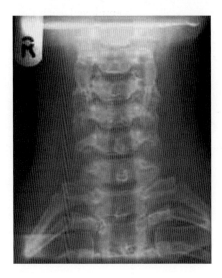

Example of
antero-posterior
cervical spine
radiograph

CERVICAL SPINE – LATERAL ERECT

Position of Patient and Image Receptor

- The patient stands or sits with either shoulder against the image receptor.
- The median sagittal plane should be adjusted such that it is parallel with the image receptor.
- The head should be flexed or extended such that the angle of the mandible is not superimposed over the upper anterior cervical vertebra or the occipital bone does not obscure the posterior arch of the atlas.
- To aid immobilization, the patient should stand with the feet slightly apart and with the shoulder resting against the image receptor stand.
- In order to demonstrate the lower cervical vertebra, the shoulders should be depressed. This can be achieved by asking the patient to relax their shoulders downwards. The process can be aided by asking the patient to hold a weight in each hand (if they are capable) and making the exposure on arrested expiration.

Direction and Centring of X-ray Beam

- The horizontal central ray is centred to a point vertically below the mastoid process at the level of the prominence of the thyroid cartilage.
- An FRD of 150 cm should be used to reduce magnification.

Essential Image Characteristics

- The whole of the cervical spine and upper part of TV1 should be included.
- The mandible or occipital bone should not obscure any part of the upper vertebra.
- Angles of the mandible and the lateral portions of the floor of the posterior cranial fossa should be superimposed.
- Soft tissues of the neck should be included.

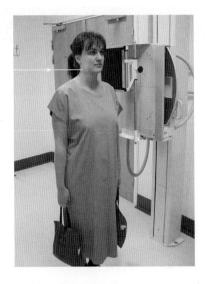

Positioning for lateral
cervical spine

Floor of posterior
cranial fossa
(occipital bone)

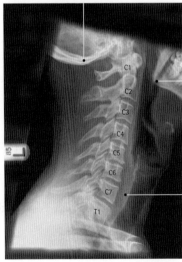

C1

C2

C3

C4

C5

C6

C7

T1

Angle of
mandible

Prevertebral
soft tissue

Example of lateral
cervical spine
radiograph

57

CERVICAL SPINE – ANTERO-POSTERIOR C1–C2 'OPEN MOUTH'

Position of Patient and Image Receptor

- The patient lies supine on the Bucky table or, if erect positioning is preferred, sits or stands with the posterior aspect of the head and shoulders against the vertical Bucky.
- The median sagittal plane is adjusted to coincide with the midline of the image receptor, such that it is at right-angles to it.
- The neck is extended, if possible, such that a line joining the tip of the mastoid process and the inferior border of the upper incisors is at right-angles to the image receptor. This will superimpose the upper incisors and the occipital bone, thus allowing clear visualization of the area of interest.
- The image receptor is centred at the level of the mastoid process.

Direction and Centring of X-ray Beam

- Direct the perpendicular central ray along the midline to the centre of the open mouth.
- If the patient is unable to flex the neck and attain the position described above, then the beam must be angled, typically 5 to 10 degrees cranially or caudally, to superimpose the upper incisors on the occipital bone.
- The image receptor position may have to be altered slightly to allow the image to be centred after beam angulation.

Essential Image Characteristics

- The inferior border of the upper central incisors should be superimposed over the occipital bone.
- The whole of the articulation between the atlas and the axis must be demonstrated clearly.
- Ideally, the whole of the dens, the lateral masses of the atlas and as much of the axis as possible should be included within the image.

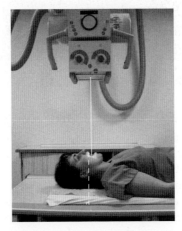

Positioning for antero-posterior
C1–C2

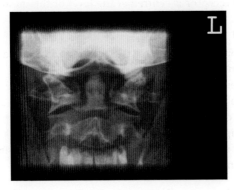

Correctly positioned radiograph

CERVICAL SPINE – LATERAL 'SWIMMER'S'

Position of Patient and Image Receptor

- This projection is usually carried out with the patient supine on a trauma trolley. The trolley is positioned adjacent to the vertical Bucky, with the patient's median sagittal plane parallel with the image receptor.
- The arm nearest the image receptor is folded over the head, with the humerus as close to the trolley top as the patient can manage. The arm and shoulder nearest the X-ray tube are depressed as far as possible.
- The shoulders are now separated vertically.
- The Bucky should be raised or lowered, such that the line of the vertebrae coincides with the middle of the image receptor.
- This projection can also be undertaken with the patient erect, either standing or sitting.

Direction and Centring of X-ray Beam

- The horizontal central ray is directed to the midline of the Bucky at a level just above the shoulder remote from the image receptor.

Essential Image Characteristics

- It is imperative to ensure that the C7–T1 junction has been included on the image. It is therefore useful to include an anatomical landmark within the image, e.g. atypical CV2. This will make it possible to count down the vertebrae and ensure that the junction has been imaged.

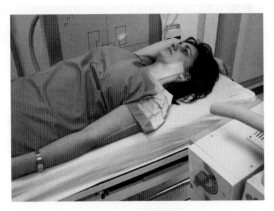

Positioning for 'swimmer's' projection

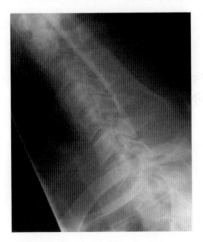

Example of 'swimmer's' projection

CERVICAL SPINE – LATERAL SUPINE

Position of Patient and Image Receptor

- This projection is normally undertaken on trauma patients who arrive in the supine position.
- It is vitally important for the patient to depress the shoulders as much as possible (assuming no other injuries would contraindicate this).
- The receptor can be either supported vertically or placed in the erect receptor holder, with the top of the receptor at the same level as the top of the ear.
- To further depress the shoulders, one or two suitably qualified individuals can apply caudal traction to the arms. NB: Refer to departmental local rules for staff working within a controlled area.

Direction and Centring of X-ray Beam

- The horizontal central ray is centred to a point vertically below the mastoid process at the level of the prominence of the thyroid cartilage.

Essential Image Characteristics

- The whole of the cervical spine should be included, from the atlanto-occipital joints to the top of the first thoracic vertebra.
- Soft tissues of the neck should be included.
- The contrast should produce a grey scale sufficient to demonstrate soft tissue and bony detail.
- Failure to demonstrate C7–T1: if the patient's shoulders are depressed fully, then the application of traction will normally show half to one extra vertebra inferiorly. Should the cervical thoracic junction still remain undemonstrated, then a swimmer's lateral, oblique projection or CT should be considered.

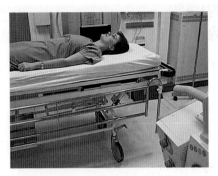

Positioning for lateral supine

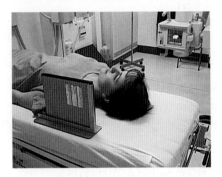

The image receptor may be supported as shown

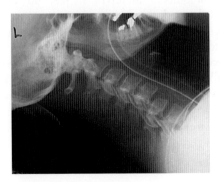

Fracture dislocation C5–C6

CERVICAL SPINE – POSTERIOR OBLIQUE

Position of Patient and Image Receptor

- The patient stands or sits with the posterior aspect of their head and shoulders against the image receptor.
- The median sagittal plane of the trunk is rotated through 45 degrees for right and left sides in turn.
- The head can be rotated so that the median sagittal plane of the head is parallel to the receptor, thus avoiding superimposition of the mandible on the vertebra.
- The receptor is centred at the prominence of the thyroid cartilage.

Direction and Centring of X-ray Beam

- The beam is angled 15 degrees cranially from the horizontal and the central ray is directed to the middle of the neck on the side nearest the tube.

Essential Image Characteristics

- The intervertebral foramina should be demonstrated clearly.
- C1–T1 should be included within the image.
- The mandible and the occipital bone should be clear of the vertebrae.

Additional Considerations

- In trauma cases the projection may be undertaken supine with the beam angled 30–45 degrees to the median sagittal plane. The image receptor should be displaced to one side to account for the beam angulation and no grid should be used as a grid 'cut off' artefact will result.

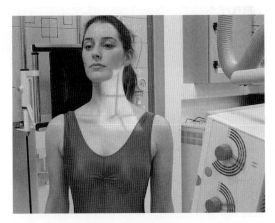

Positioning for oblique cervical spine

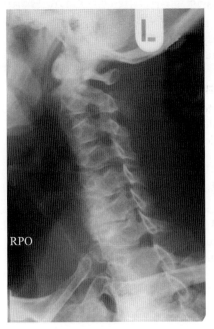

Example of oblique cervical spine image

CERVICAL SPINE – FLEXION AND EXTENSION

Position of Patient and Image Receptor

- The patient is positioned as for the lateral basic or lateral supine projections; however, erect positioning is more convenient. The patient is asked to flex the neck and to tuck the chin in towards the chest as far as is possible.
- The patient is then asked to extend the neck by raising the chin as far as possible.
- The image receptor is centred to the mid-cervical region and may have to be placed transversely for the lateral in flexion, depending on the degree of movement and the image receptor used.
- If imaged supine, the neck can be flexed by placing pads under the neck and head. Extension of the neck can be achieved by placing pillows under the patient's shoulders.

Direction and Centring of X-ray Beam

- Direct the central ray horizontally towards the mid-cervical region (C4).
- The image should include the cervical vertebrae, atlanto-occipital joints and the spinous processes.

Essential Image Characteristics

- The final image should include all the cervical vertebrae, including the atlanto-occipital joints, the spinous processes and the soft tissues of the neck.

Additional Considerations

- Refer to local protocols for the need for medical supervision when moving the spine or removing immobilization collars if undertaking these examinations on patients with suspected trauma or an unstable spine.

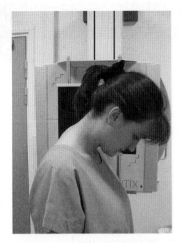

Flexion

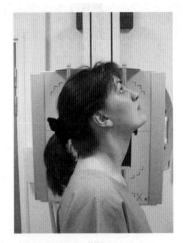

Extension

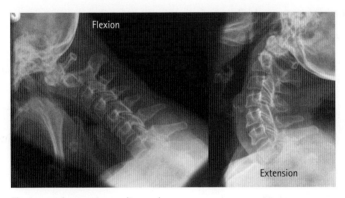

Flexion and extension radiographs

CHEST – POSTERO-ANTERIOR

Position of Patient and Image Receptor

- The patient faces the image receptor, with the feet slightly apart for stability and chin extended and placed on the top of the image receptor.
- The median sagittal plane is adjusted at right-angles to the middle of the image receptor. The dorsal aspects of the hands are placed behind and below the hips, with the elbows brought forward and the shoulders rotated anteriorly and pressed downward in contact with the image receptor.
- For patients with reduced mobility an alternative is to allow the arms to encircle the image receptor.

Direction and Centring of X-ray Beam

- The horizontal central beam is directed at right-angles to the image receptor at the level of the eighth thoracic vertebrae (i.e. spinous process of T7 – found by using the inferior angle of the scapula).
- Exposure is made in full normal arrested inspiration.
- An FRD of 180 cm should be used to minimize magnification.

Essential Image Characteristics

- Full lung fields with the scapulae projected laterally away from the lung fields and clavicles symmetrical and equidistant from the spinous processes.
- Sufficient inspiration – visualizing either six ribs anteriorly or 10 ribs posteriorly.
- The costophrenic angles, diaphragm, mediastinum, lung markings and heart should be defined sharply.

Additional Considerations

- An expiration radiograph may be obtained to demonstrate a small apical pneumothorax.

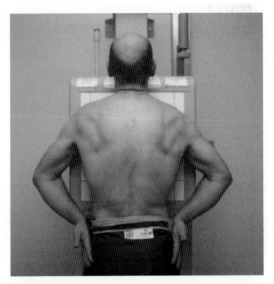

Positioning for postero-anterior chest

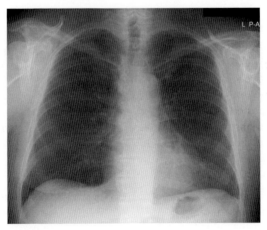

Example of postero-anterior chest radiograph

CHEST – ANTERO-POSTERIOR (ERECT)

This projection is often used as an alternative when the postero-anterior projection cannot be performed due to the patient's condition. Frequently the patient is supported sitting erect on a chair.

Position of Patient and Image Receptor

- The patient sits with their back against the image receptor, with the upper edge of the image receptor above the lung apices.
- The median sagittal plane is adjusted at right-angles to the middle of the image receptor.
- Dependent on the patient's condition, the arms are extended forwards into the anatomical position and internally rotated to minimize the superimposition of the scapulae on the lung fields.

Direction and Centring of X-ray Beam

- The horizontal ray is directed first at right-angles to the image receptor and towards the sternal notch.
- The central ray is then angled until it is coincident with the middle of the image receptor. This has the effect of confining the radiation field to the image receptor, avoiding unnecessary exposure of the eyes.
- The exposure is taken on normal full inspiration.
- An FRD of at least 120 cm is essential to reduce unequal magnification of intrathoracic structures.

Essential Image Characteristics

- The image should be of comparable quality to that described for the postero-anterior chest projection.

Additional Considerations

- The heart is moved further from the image receptor, thus increasing magnification and reducing accuracy of assessment of heart size (cardiothoracic ratio (CRT)).

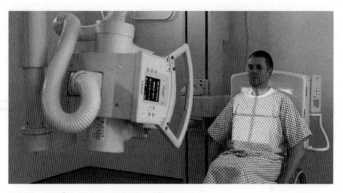

Positioning for antero-posterior chest

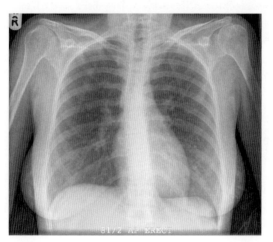

Example of antero-posterior chest radiograph

CHEST – LATERAL

Position of Patient and Image Receptor

- This projection may be undertaken with or without a grid, depending on patient size and local protocols.
- The patient is turned to bring the side under investigation in contact with the image receptor.
- The median sagittal plane is adjusted parallel to the image receptor.
- The arms are folded over the head or raised above the head to rest on a horizontal bar.
- The mid-axillary line is coincident with the middle of the image receptor, which is then is adjusted to include the apices and the lower lobes to the level of the first lumbar vertebra.

Direction and Centring of X-ray Beam

- Direct the horizontal central ray at right-angles to the middle of the image receptor at the mid-axillary line.

Essential Image Characteristics

- The image should include the apices and costophrenic angles and lung margins anteriorly and posteriorly.
- Image processing should be optimized to visualize the heart and lung tissue, with particular regard to any lesions if appropriate.

Additional Considerations

- The projection is useful to confirm position and size of a lesion suspected on the initial projection or the position of leads post pacemaker insertion.
- However, it is not a routine examination because of the additional patient dose and the increasing use of computed tomography to examine the thorax.

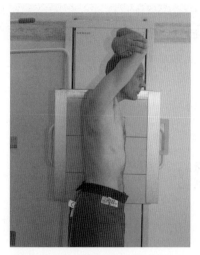

Positioning for lateral chest

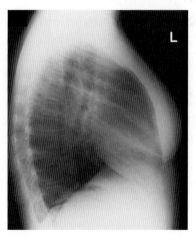

Example of lateral chest radiograph

CHEST – SUPINE (ANTERO-POSTERIOR)

This projection is usually only utilized when the patient is unable to sit up on a bed or trolley.

Position of Patient and Image Receptor

- With assistance, an image receptor is carefully positioned under the patient's chest with the upper edge of the image receptor above the lung apices.
- The median sagittal plane is adjusted at right-angles to the middle of the image receptor.
- The arms are rotated laterally and supported by the side of the trunk. The head is supported on a pillow, with the chin slightly raised. The pelvis is checked for rotation.

Direction and Centring of X-ray Beam

- As described for the sitting antero-posterior position (page 70).

Essential Image Characteristics

- The image quality may be compromised due to the patient's condition and the drawbacks of this technique; however, the apices, lateral lung margins and bases should be visualized with optimum image processing and resolution with no evidence of rotation.

Additional Considerations

- Maximum lung demonstration is lost due to the absence of the gravity effect of the abdominal organs, which is present in the erect position.
- A pleural effusion or a pneumothorax is not as well demonstrated compared with the erect projections.
- An FRD of at least 120 cm is essential to reduce unequal magnification of intrathoracic structures.

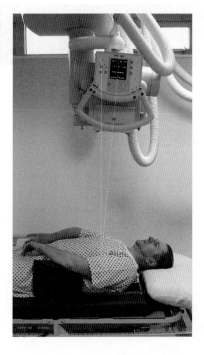

Positioning for supine chest

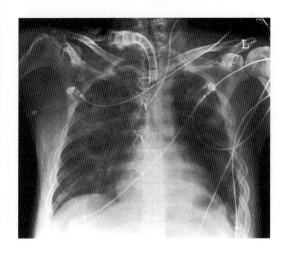

Example of supine
chest radiograph

CHEST – MOBILE/TROLLEY (ANTERO-POSTERIOR)

Ward radiography should only be performed when necessary, by properly justifying the examination and checking previous images for consistency.

Position of Patient and Image Receptor

- Where possible, the patient should be examined in an erect position, however this may not be achievable due to the patient's condition.
- The image receptor is supported behind the back of the patient, using pads/pillows as required.
- It is very important to avoid/minimize any rotation, which can make interpretation difficult.

Direction and Centring of X-ray Beam

- As described for the sitting antero-posterior position (page 70).

Essential Image Characteristics

- As described for the supine chest position (page 74).

Additional Considerations

The radiographer needs to consider issues such as:
- careful identification of the patient
- moving and handling issues
- care when handling any patient devices such as drains or lines
- infection control
- radiation protection: use of lead rubber aprons; responsibility for the controlled area and protecting patients via careful selection of exposure factors, collimation and lead backstops where necessary
- good communication with nursing staff
- it is good practice to annotate the image with information to assist with consistency of results. This may include the date, time, exposure, patient position and FRD.

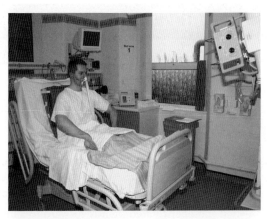

Positioning for mobile chest

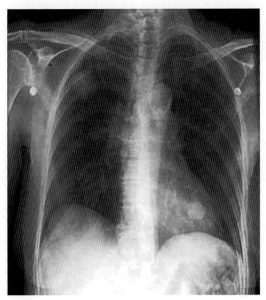

Example of mobile chest radiograph demonstrating
metastatic spread

CLAVICLE – POSTERO-ANTERIOR

Although the clavicle is demonstrated on the antero-posterior 'survey' image, it is desirable to have the clavicle as close to the image receptor as possible to give optimum bony detail.

Position of Patient and Image Receptor

- The patient sits or stands facing the image receptor.
- The patient's position is adjusted so that the middle of the clavicle is in the centre of the image receptor.
- The patient's head is turned away from the side being examined and the affected shoulder rotated slightly forward to allow the affected clavicle to be brought into close contact with the image receptor.

Direction and Centring of X-ray Beam

- The horizontal central ray is directed to the centre of the clavicle with the beam collimated to the clavicle.

Essential Image Characteristics

- The entire length of the clavicle should be included on the image.
- The lateral end of the clavicle will be demonstrated clear of the thoracic cage.
- There should be no foreshortening of the clavicle.
- The exposure should demonstrate both the medial and the lateral ends of the clavicle.

Notes

- Exposure is made on arrested respiration to eliminate patient movement.

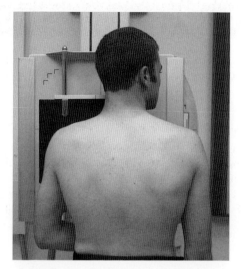

Positioning for postero-anterior clavicle

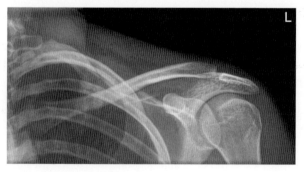

Radiograph for postero-anterior clavicle

CLAVICLE – INFERO-SUPERIOR

In cases of acute injury, it is more comfortable for the patient to be examined in the erect position.

Position of Patient and Image Receptor

- The patient sits or stands facing the image X-ray tube.
- The patient's position is adjusted so that the middle of the clavicle is in the centre of the image receptor.

Direction and Centring of X-ray Beam

- The central ray is angled 30 degrees cranially and centred to the centre of the clavicle.
- The medial end of the clavicle can be shown in greater detail by adding a 15-degree lateral angulation to the beam.

Essential Image Characteristics

- The image should demonstrate the entire length of the clavicle, including the sternoclavicular and acromioclavicular joints and should be projected clear of the thoracic cage.
- The clavicle should be horizontal.

Notes

- The 30 degrees needed to separate the clavicle from the underlying ribs can be achieved by a combination of patient positioning and central ray angulation.
- If a fracture occurs together with fracture of the upper ribs, then this implies a severe injury and may be associated with subclavian vessel damage or pneumothorax.

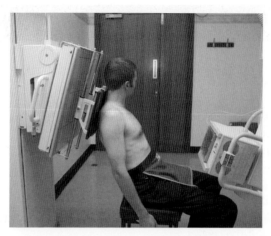

Positioning for infero-superior clavicle

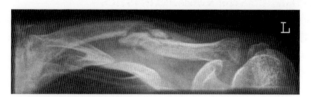

Infero-superior radiograph of fractured clavicle

COCCYX – LATERAL

Position of Patient and Image Receptor

- The patient lies on their side on the Bucky table, with the palpable coccyx in the midline of the Bucky. The arms are raised, with the hands resting on the pillow. The knees and hips are flexed slightly for stability.
- The dorsal aspect of the trunk should be at right-angles to the image receptor. This can be assessed by palpating the iliac crests or the posterior superior iliac spines. The median sagittal plane should be parallel with the Bucky.
- The image receptor is centred to coincide with the central ray at the level of the coccyx.

Direction and Centring of X-ray Beam

- Direct the central ray at right-angles to the long axis of the sacrum and towards the palpable coccyx.

Additional Considerations

- Care must be taken when using an automatic exposure control, as underexposure can easily result if the chamber is positioned slightly posterior to the coccyx.

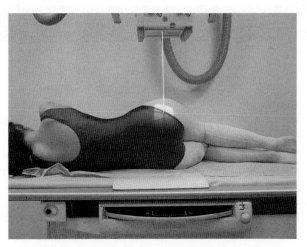

Positioning for lateral coccyx

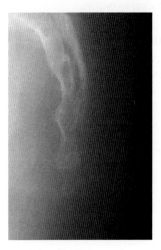

Example of lateral coccyx
radiograph

ELBOW – ANTERO-POSTERIOR

Position of Patient and Image Receptor

- The patient is seated alongside the table with the affected arm nearest to the table.
- The arm is extended fully, such that the posterior aspect of the entire limb is in contact with the tabletop and the palm of the hand is facing upwards.
- The image receptor is positioned under the elbow joint.
- The arm is adjusted such that the medial and lateral epicondyles are equidistant from the image receptor.
- The limb is immobilized using sandbags.

Direction and Centring of X-ray Beam

- The vertical central ray is centred through the joint space 2.5 cm distal to the point midway between the medial and lateral epicondyles of the humerus.

Essential Image Characteristics

- The central ray must pass through the joint space at 90 degrees to the humerus to provide a satisfactory view of the joint space.
- The image should demonstrate the distal third of humerus and the proximal third of the radius and ulna.

Notes

- When the patient is unable to extend the elbow to 90 degrees, a modified technique is used for the antero-posterior projection.
- If the limb cannot be moved, two projections at right-angles to each other can be taken by keeping the limb in the same position and rotating the X-ray tube through 90 degrees.

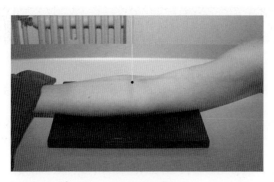

Positioning for antero-posterior elbow

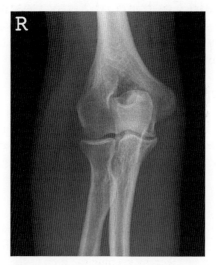

Antero-posterior elbow radiograph

ELBOW – ANTERO-POSTERIOR ALTERNATE PROJECTIONS FOR TRAUMA

These projections may be useful in cases of trauma when the patient is unable to extend the elbow joint.

Position of Patient and Imaging Receptor

This is fundamentally the same as an antero-posterior elbow and the same for all projections; however, either the upper arm or forearm is in contact with the image receptor depending on the area of interest.

- Forearm in contact with image receptor for suspected radial head and olecranon fractures.
- Upper arm in contact with image receptor for suspected supracondylar fractures.
- Axial projection when the patient cannot extend their arm to any extent.

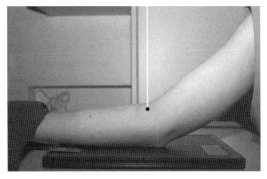

Forearm in contact with receptor

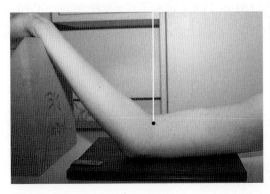

Upper arm in contact with receptor

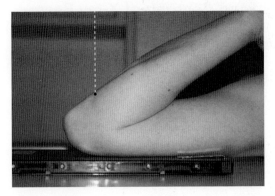

Axial projection

ELBOW – LATERAL

Position of Patient and Image Receptor

- The patient is seated alongside the table, with the affected side nearest to the table.
- The elbow is flexed to 90 degrees and the palm of the hand is rotated so that it is at 90 degrees to the tabletop.
- The shoulder is lowered so that it is at the same height as the elbow and wrist, such that the medial aspect of the entire arm is in contact with the tabletop.
- The image receptor is placed under the patient's elbow, with its centre to the elbow joint.
- The limb is immobilized using sandbags.

Direction and Centring of X-ray Beam

- The vertical central ray is centred over the lateral epicondyle of the humerus.

Essential Image Characteristics

- The central ray must pass through the joint space at 90 degrees to the humerus, i.e. the epicondyles should be superimposed.
- The image should demonstrate the distal third of humerus and the proximal third of the radius and ulna.

Notes

- Care should be taken when a supracondylar fracture of the humerus is suspected. In such cases, no attempt should be made to extend the elbow joint, and a modified technique must be employed.

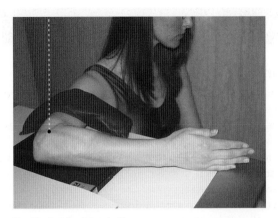

Positioning for lateral elbow

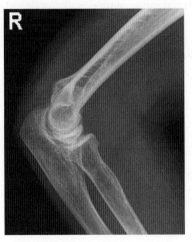

Lateral radiograph of the elbow

FACIAL BONES – OCCIPITO-MENTAL

Position of Patient and Image Receptor

- The projection is best performed erect with the patient seated facing the image receptor (a grid/Bucky should be used).
- The head is then adjusted to bring the orbito-meatal baseline to an angle of 45 degrees.
- The horizontal central line of the image receptor should be level with the lower orbital margins and the median sagittal plane should coincide with its vertical central line.
- Ensure that the median sagittal plane is at right-angles to the image receptor by checking the outer canthi of the eyes and the external auditory meatuses are equidistant.

Direction and Centring of X-ray Beam

- The central ray should be perpendicular and central to the image receptor before positioning commences (ensure the X-ray tube and Bucky are at the same height as the patient's head).
- To check that the beam is centred properly, the cross-lines on the Bucky or cassette holder should coincide with the patient's anterior nasal spine.
- Ensure the tube is recentred to the middle of the image receptor if it is moved during positioning.

Essential Image Characteristics

- The petrous ridges must appear below the floors of the maxillary sinuses.
- There should be no rotation. This can be checked by ensuring that the distance from the lateral orbital wall to the outer skull margins is equidistant on both sides (marked a and b on the image opposite).

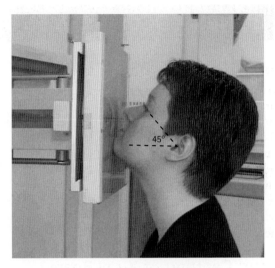

Positioning for occipito-mental projection

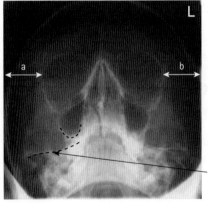

Petrous ridges just below inferior margin of maxillary sinus

Example of occipito-mental radiograph

FACIAL BONES – OCCIPITO-MENTAL 30°↓

Position of Patient and Image Receptor

- The projection is best performed erect with the patient seated facing the image receptor (a grid/Bucky should be used).
- The head is then adjusted to bring the orbito-meatal baseline to an angle of 45 degrees.
- The horizontal central line of the image receptor should be level with the symphysis menti and the median sagittal plane should coincide with its vertical central line.
- Ensure that the median sagittal plane is at right-angles to the image receptor by checking the outer canthi of the eyes and the external auditory meatuses are equidistant.

Direction and Centring of X-ray Beam

- The central ray is angled 30 degrees caudally and centred along the midline, such that the central ray passes through the lower orbital margins and exits at the symphysis menti. This should coincide with the centre of the image receptor.
- To check that the beam is centred properly, the cross-lines on the Bucky should coincide approximately with the upper symphysis menti region (this may vary with anatomical differences between patients).

Essential Image Characteristics

- The floors of the orbit will be clearly visible through the maxillary sinuses, and the lower orbital margin should be demonstrated clearly.
- There should be no rotation. This is checked by ensuring the distance from the lateral orbital wall to the outer skull margins is equidistant on both sides.

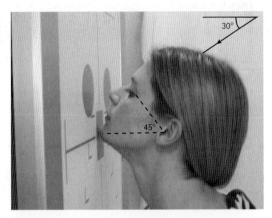

Positioning for occipito-mental (OM)30°↓ projection

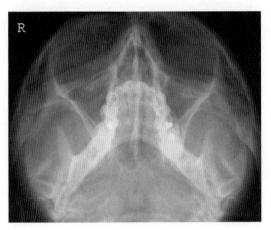

Example of occipito-mental (OM)30°↓ radiograph

FEMUR – ANTERO-POSTERIOR

Position of Patient and Image Receptor

- The patient lies supine on the X-ray table, with both legs extended.
- The affected limb is rotated to centralize the patella over the femur.
- Sandbags are placed below the knee to help maintain the position.
- The image receptor is positioned in the Bucky tray immediately under the limb, adjacent to the posterior aspect of the thigh to include both the hip and the knee joints.
- Alternatively, the image receptor is positioned directly under the limb, against the posterior aspect of the thigh to include the knee joint.

Direction and Centring of X-ray Beam

- Centre to the middle of the image receptor, with the vertical central ray at 90 degrees to an imaginary line joining both femoral condyles.

Essential Image Characteristics

The hip and knee joints should both be included on the image where possible.

Additional Considerations

- In suspected fractures, the limb must not be rotated.
- The knee and hip joints should be included on the image. If this is impossible to achieve, then the joint nearest the site of injury should be included.
- If the distal femur is the focus of attention, and the effects of scatter are not of pressing concern, the image receptor can be placed directly under the femur.

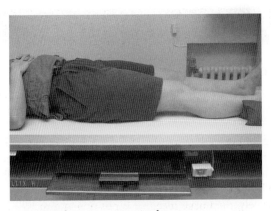

Positioning for antero-posterior femur

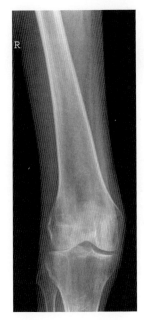

Antero-posterior femur
'knee up'

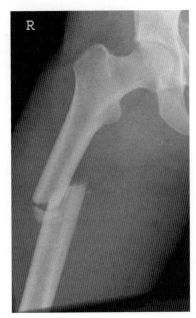

Antero-posterior femur 'hip down'

FEMUR – LATERAL

Position of Patient and Image Receptor

- From the antero-posterior position, the patient rotates onto the affected side, and the knee is slightly flexed.
- The pelvis is rotated backwards to separate the thighs.
- The position of the limb is then adjusted to vertically superimpose the femoral condyles.
- Pads are used to support the opposite limb behind the one being examined.
- The image receptor is positioned in the Bucky tray under the lateral aspect of the thigh to include the knee joint and as much of the femur as possible.
- Alternatively, the image receptor is positioned directly under the limb, against the lateral aspect of the thigh, to include the knee joint.

Direction and Centring of X-ray Beam

- Centre to the middle of the image receptor, with the vertical central ray parallel to the imaginary line joining the femoral condyles.

Essential Image Characteristics

- The image should show from the 'knee up' to the proximal third of the femur.

Additional Considerations

- In some slim patients, it is possible to demonstrate up to the femoral head; however, a separate image of this proximal region may be needed if the entire length of the femur is required to be seen.

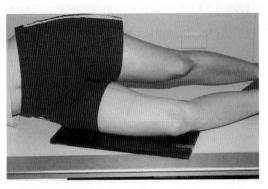

Positioning for lateral femur

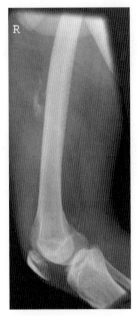

Lateral femur: 'knee up'

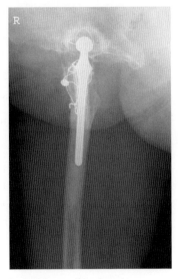

Lateral femur: 'hip down'
demonstrating a hip prosthesis

FINGERS – DORSI-PALMAR

Position of Patient and Image Receptor

- The patient is positioned seated alongside the table as for a dorsi-palmar projection of the hand.
- The forearm is pronated with the anterior (palmar) aspect of the finger(s) in contact with the image receptor.
- The finger(s) are extended and separated.
- A sandbag is placed across the dorsal surface of the wrist for immobilization.

Direction and Centring of X-ray Beam

- The vertical central ray is centred over the proximal interphalangeal joint of the affected finger.

Essential Image Characteristics

- The image should include the fingertips, including soft tissues.
- It is necessary to include adjacent finger(s), i.e. second and third or fourth and fifth to aid identification of relevant anatomy.

Additional Considerations

- The image should include the fingertip and the distal third of the metacarpal bone.

Notes

- It is common practice to obtain two projections, a dorsi-palmar and a lateral.

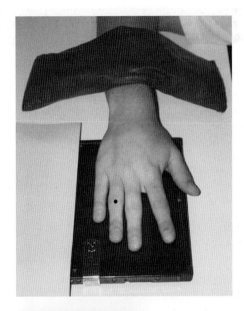

Positioning for
dorsi-palmar
finger

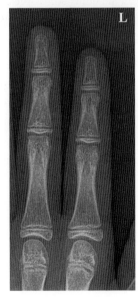

Dorsi-palmar radiograph of the
index and middle fingers

FINGERS – LATERAL INDEX AND MIDDLE FINGERS

Position of Patient and Image Receptor

- The patient is seated alongside the table with the arm abducted and medially rotated to bring the lateral aspect of the index finger into contact with the image receptor.
- The raised forearm is supported.
- The index finger is fully extended and the middle finger slightly flexed to avoid superimposition.
- The middle finger is supported on a non-opaque pad.
- The remaining fingers are fully flexed into the palm of the hand and held there by the thumb.

Direction and Centring of X-ray Beam

- The vertical central ray is centred over the proximal interphalangeal joint of the affected finger.

Essential Image Characteristics

- The image should include the fingertip and the distal third of the metacarpal bone.

Additional Considerations

- Scleroderma (one cause of Raynaud's disease) causes wasting and calcification of the soft tissue of the finger pulp.
- Chip fracture of the base of the dorsal aspect of the distal phalanx is associated with avulsion of the insertion of the extensor digitorum tendon, leading to the mallet finger deformity.
- In cases of severe trauma, when the fingers cannot be flexed, it may be necessary to take a lateral projection of all the fingers superimposed, as for the lateral projection of the hand, but centring over the proximal interphalangeal joint of the index finger.

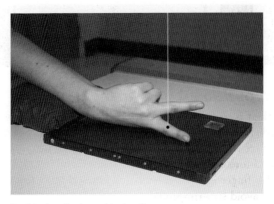

Positioning for lateral index finger

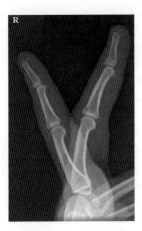

Lateral radiograph of index
and middle fingers

FINGERS – LATERAL RING AND LITTLE FINGERS

Position of Patient and Image Receptor

- The patient is seated alongside the table with the palm of the hand at right-angles to the table and the medial aspect of the little finger in contact with the image receptor.
- The affected finger is extended and the remaining fingers are fully flexed into the palm of the hand and held there by the thumb in order to prevent superimposition.
- It may be necessary to support the ring finger on a non-opaque pad to ensure that it is parallel to the image receptor.

Direction and Centring of X-ray Beam

- The vertical central ray is centred over the proximal interphalangeal joint of the affected finger.

Essential Image Characteristics

- The image should include the tip of the finger and the distal third of the metacarpal bone.

Additional Considerations

- Scleroderma (one cause of Raynaud's disease) causes wasting and calcification of the soft tissue of the finger pulp.
- Chip fracture of the base of the dorsal aspect of the distal phalanx is associated with avulsion of the insertion of the extensor digitorum tendon, leading to the mallet finger deformity.
- In cases of severe trauma, when the fingers cannot be flexed, it may be necessary to take a lateral projection of all the fingers superimposed, as for the lateral projection of the hand, but centring over the proximal interphalangeal joint of the index finger.

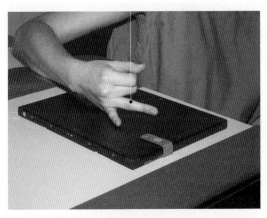

Positioning for ring and little fingers

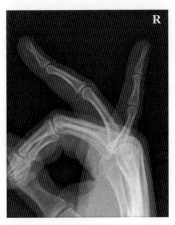

Lateral radiograph of ring and little fingers

FOOT – DORSI-PLANTAR

Position of Patient and Image Receptor

- The patient is seated on the X-ray table, supported if necessary, with the affected hip and knee flexed.
- The plantar aspect of the affected foot is placed on the image receptor and the lower leg is supported in the vertical position by the other knee.
- Alternatively, the image receptor can be raised on a 15-degree foam pad for ease of positioning.

Direction and Centring of X-ray Beam

- The central ray is directed over the cuboid-navicular joint, midway between the palpable navicular tuberosity and the tuberosity of the fifth metatarsal.
- The X-ray tube is angled 15 degrees cranially when the image receptor is flat on the table.
- The X-ray tube is vertical when the image receptor is raised on a 15-degree pad.

Essential Image Characteristics

- The tarsal and tarsometatarsal joints should be demonstrated when the whole foot is examined.
- The kVp selected should reduce the difference in subject contrast between the thickness of the toes and the tarsus to give a uniform radiographic contrast over the range of foot densities.

Additional Considerations

- A wedge filter can be used to compensate for the difference in tissue thickness.

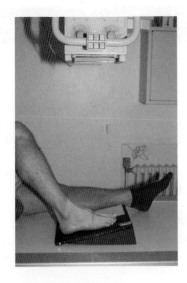

Positioning for
dorsi-plantar foot

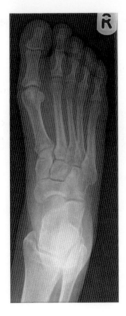

Example of dorsi-plantar foot

FOOT – DORSI-PLANTAR OBLIQUE

Position of Patient and Image Receptor

- From the basic dorsi-plantar position, the affected limb is allowed to lean medially to bring the plantar surface of the foot approximately 30–45 degrees to the image receptor.
- A non-opaque angled pad is placed under the foot to maintain the position, with the opposite limb acting as a support.

Direction and Centring of X-ray Beam

- The vertical central ray is directed over the cuboid-navicular joint.

Essential Image Characteristics

- The dorsi-plantar oblique should demonstrate the inter-tarsal and tarsometatarsal joints.
- The projection should allow the alignment of the metatarsals with the distal row of the tarsus to be assessed.
- The base of the fifth metatarsal should be clearly seen.

Additional Considerations

- Be aware of the location of possible accessory ossicles around the foot. Do not confuse these with avulsion fractures, which are generally not as rounded in appearance.
- The appearance of the unfused apophysis at the base of the fifth metatarsal in children/adolescents is variable and frequently causes confusion. (As a rule of thumb, a fracture is transverse and an apophysis is parallel to the base of the fifth metatarsal.)

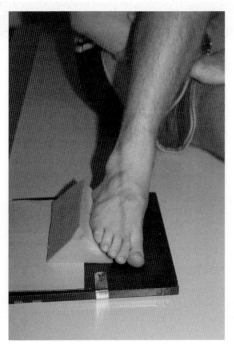

Positioning for dorsi-plantar oblique

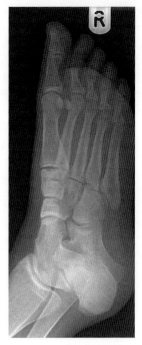

Example of dorsi-plantar
oblique radiograph

FOOT – LATERAL ERECT

Position of Patient and Image Receptor

- The patient stands on a low platform with the image receptor placed vertically between the feet.
- The feet are brought close together. The weight of the patient's body is distributed equally.
- To help maintain the position, the patient should rest their forearms on a convenient vertical support, e.g. the vertical Bucky.

Direction and Centring of X-ray Beam

- The horizontal central ray is directed towards the tubercle of the fifth metatarsal.

Essential Image Characteristics

- The image should include the distal phalanges and calcaneum.
- The ankle joint and soft tissue margins of the plantar aspect of the foot should be included.
- The longitudinal arches of the feet should be clearly demonstrated.

Additional Considerations

- Frequently both feet are imaged for comparison.
- Images should be labelled as 'standing' or 'weight bearing'.

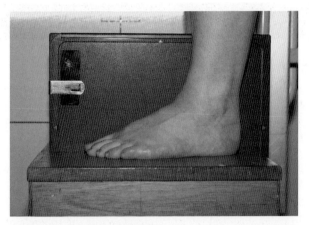

Positioning for lateral erect foot

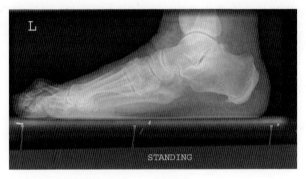

Example of lateral erect foot radiograph

FOREARM – ANTERO-POSTERIOR

Position of Patient and Image Receptor

- The patient is seated alongside the table, with the affected side nearest to the table.
- The arm is abducted and the elbow joint is fully extended, with the supinated forearm resting on the table.
- The shoulder is lowered to the same level as the elbow joint.
- The image receptor is placed under the forearm to include the wrist joint and the elbow joint.
- The arm is adjusted such that the radial and ulnar styloid processes and the medial and lateral epicondyles are equidistant from the image receptor.
- The lower end of the humerus and the hand are immobilized using sandbags.

Direction and Centring of X-ray Beam

- The vertical central ray is centred in the midline of the forearm to a point midway between the wrist and elbow joints.

Essential Image Characteristics

- Both the elbow and the wrist joint must be demonstrated on the radiograph.
- Both joints should be seen in the true antero-posterior position, with the radial and ulnar styloid processes and the epicondyles of the humerus equidistant from the image receptor.

Notes

- The postero-anterior projection of the forearm with the wrist pronated is not satisfactory because, in this projection, the radius is superimposed over the ulna for part of its length.

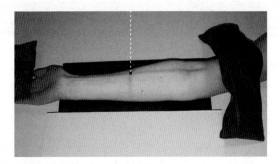

Positioning for antero-posterior forearm

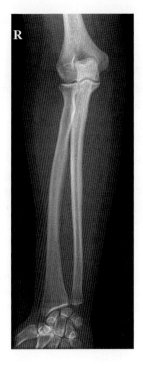

Example of antero-posterior
forearm radiograph

FOREARM – LATERAL

Position of Patient and Image Receptor

- From the antero-posterior position, the elbow is flexed to 90 degrees.
- The humerus is internally rotated to 90 degrees to bring the medial aspect of the upper arm, elbow, forearm, wrist and hand into contact with the table.
- The image receptor is placed under the forearm to include the wrist joint and the elbow joint.
- The arm is adjusted such that the radial and ulnar styloid processes and the medial and lateral epicondyles are superimposed.
- The lower end of the humerus and the hand are immobilized using sandbags.

Direction and Centring of X-ray Beam

- The vertical central ray is centred in the midline of the forearm to a point midway between the wrist and elbow joints.

Essential Image Characteristics

- Both the elbow and the wrist joint must be demonstrated on the image.
- Both joints should be seen in the true lateral position, with the radial and ulnar styloid processes and the epicondyles of the humerus superimposed.

Notes

- In trauma cases, it may be impossible to move the arm into the positions described, and a modified technique may need to be employed to ensure that diagnostic images are obtained.
- If the limb cannot be moved through 90 degrees, then a horizontal beam should be used.
- Both joints should be included on each image.
- No attempt should be made to rotate the patient's hand.

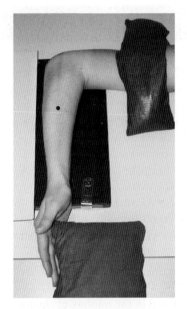

Positioning for lateral forearm

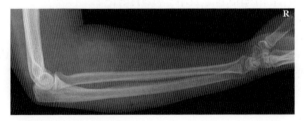

Lateral forearm radiograph

113

HAND – DORSI-PALMAR

Position of Patient and Image Receptor

- The patient is seated alongside the table with the affected arm nearest to the table.
- The forearm is pronated and placed on the table with the palmar surface of the hand in contact with the image receptor.
- The fingers are separated and extended but relaxed to ensure that they remain in contact with the image receptor.
- The wrist is adjusted so that the radial and ulna styloid processes are equidistant from the image receptor.
- A sandbag is placed over the lower forearm for immobilization.

Direction and Centring of X-ray Beam

- The vertical central ray is centred over the head of the third metacarpal.

Essential Image Characteristics

- The image should demonstrate all the phalanges, including the soft-tissue fingertips, the carpal and metacarpal bones, and the distal end of the radius and ulna.
- The interphalangeal and metacarpo-phalangeal and carpo-metacarpal joints should be demonstrated clearly.
- No rotation.

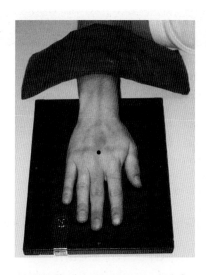

Positioning for
dorsi-palmar hand

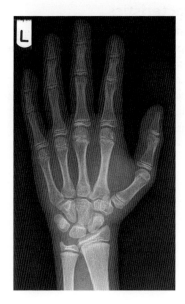

Example of a dorsi-palmar
hand radiograph

HAND – DORSI-PALMAR OBLIQUE

Position of Patient and Image Receptor

- From the basic dorsi-palmar position, the hand is externally rotated 45 degrees with the fingers extended in contact with the image receptor.
- The fingers should be separated slightly and the hand supported on a 45-degree non-opaque pad.
- A sandbag is placed over the lower end of the forearm for immobilization.

Direction and Centring of X-ray Beam

- The vertical central ray is centred over the head of the fifth metacarpal.
- The tube is then angled so that the central ray passes through the head of the third metacarpal, enabling a reduction in the size of the field.

Essential Image Characteristics

- The image should demonstrate all the phalanges, including the soft-tissue of the fingertips, the carpal and metacarpal bones, and the distal end of the radius and ulna.
- The exposure factors selected must produce a density and contrast that optimally demonstrate joint detail.
- The heads of the metacarpals should not be superimposed.

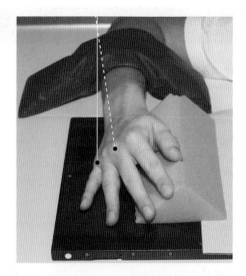

Positioning of
dorsi-palmar oblique
hand

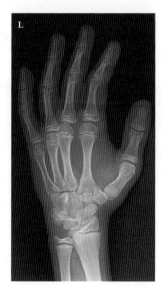

Radiograph of dorsi-palmar oblique
hand

HAND – LATERAL

Position of Patient and Image Receptor

- From the postero-anterior position, the hand is externally rotated 90 degrees.
- The palm of the hand is perpendicular to the image receptor, with the fingers extended and the thumb abducted and supported parallel to the image receptor on a non-opaque pad.
- The radial and ulnar styloid processes are superimposed.

Direction and Centring of X-ray Beam

- The vertical central ray is centred over the head of the second metacarpal.

Essential Image Characteristics

- The image should include the fingertips, including soft tissue, and the radial and ulnar styloid processes.
- The heads of the metacarpals should be superimposed. The thumb should be demonstrated clearly without superimposition of other structures.

Additional Considerations

- The hand and wrist (like the ankle and foot) have many accessory ossicles, which may trap the unwary into a false diagnosis of pathology.
- 'Boxer's fracture' of the neck of the fifth metacarpal is seen easily, but conspicuity of fractures of the bases of the metacarpals is reduced by over rotation and underexposure.

Notes

- If the projection is undertaken to identify the position of a foreign body, the kVp should be lowered to demonstrate or exclude its presence in the soft tissues and a metal marker used to demonstrate the site of entry of the foreign body.

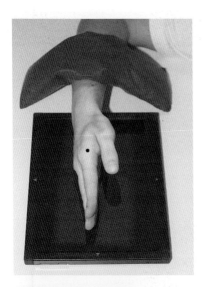

Positioning for lateral hand

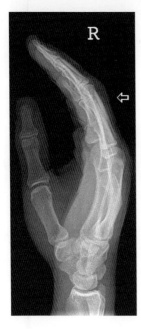

Lateral radiograph of the hand with foreign body marker. There is an old fracture of the fifth metacarpal.

HIP – ANTERO-POSTERIOR

Position of Patient and Image Receptor

The patient is positioned as described for the basic pelvis projection (see page 158).

Direction and Centring of X-ray Beam

- The vertical central ray is directed 2.5 cm distally along the perpendicular bisector of a line joining the anterior superior iliac spine and the symphysis pubis over the femoral pulse.
- The primary beam should be collimated to the area under examination and gonad protection applied where appropriate.

Essential Image Characteristics

- The image must include the upper third of the femur.
- When taken to show the positioning and integrity of an arthroplasty, the whole length of the prosthesis, including the cement, must be visualized.

Additional Considerations

- Over-rotating the limb internally will bring the greater trochanter into profile. This may be a useful supplementary projection for a suspected avulsion fracture to this bone.

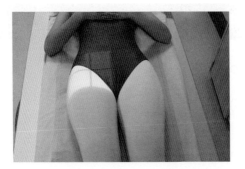

Positioning for antero-posterior hip joint

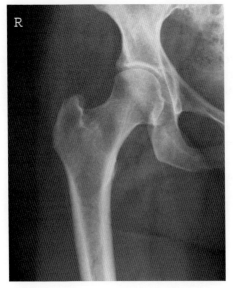

Example of antero-posterior hip radiograph

HIP – LATERAL NECK OF FEMUR (TRAUMA)

Position of Patient and Image Receptor

- The patient lies supine with the median sagittal plane perpendicular to the tabletop/trolley. A grid image receptor is positioned vertically, with the shorter edge pressed firmly against the waist, just above the iliac crest.
- If the patient is very slender, a non-opaque pad can be placed carefully under the buttock to ensure all of the essential anatomy is visualized.
- The longitudinal axis of the image receptor should be positioned parallel to the neck of femur by placing a 45-degree foam pad between the front of the image receptor and the lateral aspect of the pelvis.
- The unaffected limb is then raised until the thigh is vertical; the knee is flexed and supported by a stand.

Direction and Centring of X-ray Beam

- Centre to the affected groin, with the central ray directed horizontally and at right-angles to the image receptor to pass in line with the femoral neck. Close collimation will improve the image contrast.

Essential Image Characteristics

- The acetabulum, femoral neck, trochanters and upper third of the femur should be included.

Additional Considerations

- Modifications to the technique include using the vertical Bucky or chest stand to hold the image receptor, and turning the stretcher so its long axis is 45 degrees to the Bucky. The use of a non-grid air gap technique can also be used in slim patients.

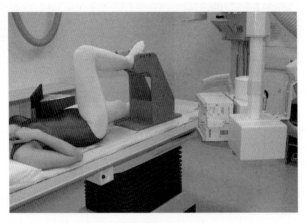

Positioning for lateral neck of femur

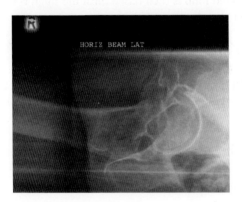

Example of lateral neck of femur radiograph showing sub-capital fracture

HIP – 'FROG LEG LATERAL'

Position of Patient and Image Receptor

- The patient lies supine on the X-ray table, with the anterior superior iliac spines equidistant from the tabletop to avoid rotation of the pelvis.
- The median sagittal plane is perpendicular to the table and coincident with the centre of the table Bucky mechanism.
- The hips and knees are flexed and the limbs rotated laterally through approximately 60 degrees. This movement separates the knees and brings the plantar aspect of the feet in contact with each other.

Direction and Centring of X-ray Beam

- Centre in the midline at the level of the femoral pulse, with the central ray perpendicular to the image receptor. Collimate to the area under examination.

Essential Image Characteristics

- The area on the image should include the upper third of both femora and the iliac crests.
- There should be evidence of properly positioned gonad protection, *unless* its presence would obscure essential anatomy.

Additional Considerations

- Often requested in conjunction with antero-posterior hips in children when Perthes' disease or slipped upper femoral epiphysis (SUFE) is suspected.
- If 60 degrees of flexion is not achievable, then it is important to apply the same degree of flexion to both hips in order not to lose symmetry.

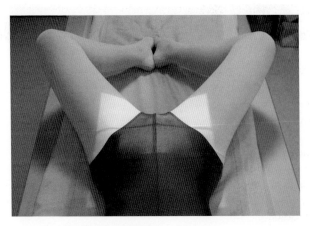

Positioning for 'frog leg lateral'

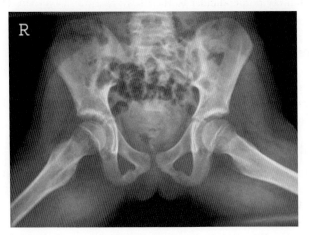

Example of 'frog leg lateral' radiograph

HUMERUS – ANTERO-POSTERIOR

Position of Patient and Image Receptor

- The image receptor is placed in an erect holder.
- The patient sits or stands with their back in contact with the image receptor.
- The patient is rotated towards the affected side to bring the posterior aspect of the shoulder, upper arm and elbow into contact with the image receptor.
- The position of the patient is adjusted to ensure that the medial and lateral epicondyles of the humerus are equidistant from the image receptor.

Direction and Centring of X-ray Beam

- The horizontal central ray is directed at right-angles to the shaft of the humerus and centred midway between the shoulder and elbow joint.

Essential Image Characteristics

- The exposure should be adjusted to ensure that the area of interest is clearly visualized.

Notes

- A type of injury commonly found in children is a fracture of the lower end of the humerus just proximal to the condyles (a supracondylar fracture). The injury is very painful and even small movements of the limb can exacerbate the injury, causing further damage to adjacent nerves and blood vessels.
- Any supporting sling should not be removed, and the patient should not be asked to extend the elbow joint or to rotate the arm or forearm.

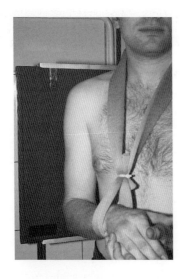

Positioning for
antero-posterior
humerus

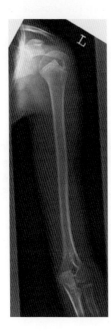

Radiograph of antero-posterior
humerus

HUMERUS – LATERAL

Position of Patient and Image Receptor

- The image receptor is placed in an erect holder.
- From the anterior position, the patient is rotated through 90 degrees until the lateral aspect of the injured arm is in contact with the image receptor.
- The patient's arm is now abducted and rotated further until the arm is just clear of the rib cage but still in contact with the image receptor.

Direction and Centring of X-ray Beam

- The horizontal central ray is directed at right-angles to the shaft of the humerus and centred midway between the shoulder and elbow joint.

Essential Image Characteristics

- The exposure should be adjusted to ensure that the area of interest is clearly visualized.

Notes

- The patient should be made as comfortable as possible to assist immobilization.
- An erect holder, or similar device, may be used to assist the patient in supporting the image receptor.
- The X-ray beam should be collimated carefully to ensure that the primary beam does not extend beyond the area of the image receptor.

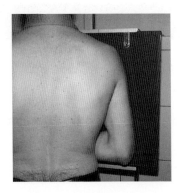

Positioning for lateral humerus

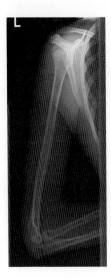

Radiograph of lateral humerus

KNEE – ANTERO-POSTERIOR

Position of Patient and Image Receptor

- For computed radiography (CR), an 18 × 24-cm image receptor is generally used.
- The patient is either supine or seated on the X-ray table, with both legs extended.
- The affected limb is rotated to centralize the patella between the femoral condyles, and sandbags are placed against the ankle to help maintain this position.
- The image receptor should be in close contact with the posterior aspect of the knee joint, with its centre level with the upper borders of the tibial condyles.

Direction and Centring of X-ray Beam

- Centre 2.5 cm below the apex of the patella through the joint space, with the central ray at 90 degrees to the long axis of the tibia.

Essential Image Characteristics

- The patella must be centralized over the femur.
- The distal third of femur and proximal third of tibia are included.

Additional Considerations

- This projection can also be undertaken in the erect position (weight bearing).

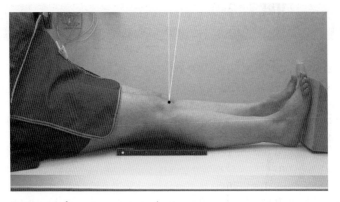

Positioning for antero-posterior knee

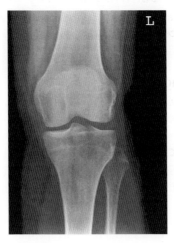

Example of antero-posterior knee
radiograph

KNEE – LATERAL

Position of Patient and Image Receptor

- The patient lies on the side to be examined, with the knee flexed at 45 or 90 degrees.
- The other limb is brought forward in front of the one being examined and supported on a sandbag.
- A sandbag is placed under the ankle of the affected side to bring the long axis of the tibia parallel to the image receptor.
- The position of the limb is now adjusted to ensure that the femoral condyles are superimposed vertically.
- The centre of the image receptor is placed level with the medial tibial condyle.

Direction and Centring of X-ray Beam

- Centre to the middle of the superior border of the medial tibial condyle, with the central ray at 90 degrees to the long axis of the tibia.

Essential Image Characteristics

- The patella should be projected clear of the femur.
- The femoral condyles should be superimposed.
- The proximal tibio-fibular joint is not clearly visible.

Additional Considerations

- A 3- to 5-degree cranial tube angulation can sometimes help superimpose the femoral condyles.
- Over-rotation = fibula is projected too posteriorly.
- Under-rotation = fibula head is hidden behind tibia.
- Identification of the *adductor tubercle* indicates the medial femoral condyle and can assist the radiographer to correct positioning faults.

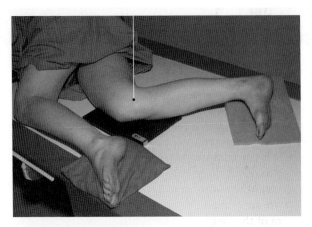

Positioning for lateral knee

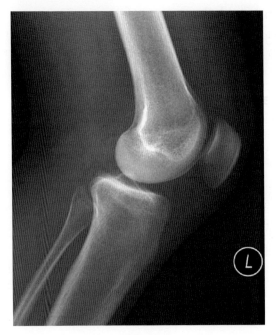

Example of lateral knee radiograph

KNEE – HORIZONTAL BEAM LATERAL (TRAUMA)

Position of Patient and Image Receptor

- For computed radiography a 24 × 30-cm image receptor is generally used.
- The patient remains on the trolley/bed, with the limb gently raised and supported on pads.
- If possible, the leg may be rotated slightly to centralize the patella between the femoral condyles.
- The image receptor is supported vertically against the medial aspect of the knee.
- The centre of the image receptor is level with the upper border of the tibial condyle.

Direction and Centring of X-ray Beam

- The horizontal central ray is directed to the upper border of the lateral tibial condyle, at 90 degrees to the long axis of the tibia.

Essential Image Characteristics

- The image should demonstrate superimposition of the femoral condyles and a clear view of the soft tissues proximally to the patella (supra-patellar pouch).

Additional Considerations

- This projection replaces the conventional lateral in all cases of gross injury and suspected fracture of the patella.
- No attempt must be made to either flex or extend the knee joint; this may cause fractures to move.
- Any rotation of the limb must be from the hip, with support given to the whole leg.
- Fluid levels and lipohaemarthrosis may be seen.

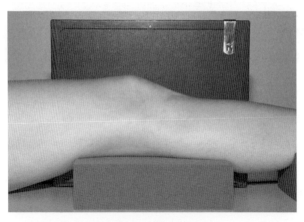

Positioning for horizontal beam lateral knee

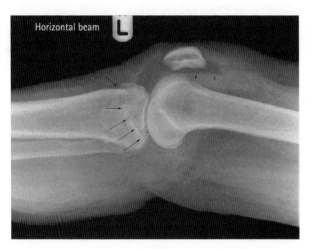

Example of horizontal beam knee radiograph showing fracture of tibial plateau (arrows) and lipohaemarthrosis (arrow heads).

KNEE – TUNNEL/INTERCONDYLAR NOTCH

Position of Patient and Image Receptor

- This projection is taken to demonstrate loose bodies within the knee joint.
- The patient is either supine or seated on the X-ray table, with the affected knee flexed to approximately 60 degrees.
- A suitable pad is placed under the knee to help maintain the position.
- The limb is rotated to centralize the patella over the femur.
- The image receptor is placed on top of the pad as close as possible to the posterior aspect of the knee and displaced towards the femur.

Direction and Centring of X-ray Beam

- Centre immediately below the apex of the patella.
- Two different tube angulations are used in relation to the long axis of the tibia: 90 degrees = posterior aspect of notch shown; 110 degrees = anterior aspect of notch shown.

Essential Image Characteristics

- The open 'notch' shape is clearly seen, demonstrating any radio-opaque loose bodies.

Additional Considerations

- Commonly only the 90-degree angulation is used.
- Take care when flexing the knee if a fracture is suspected.

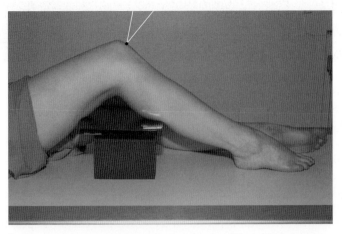

Positioning for intercondylar projection showing 90- and 110-degree beam angulations to the tibia

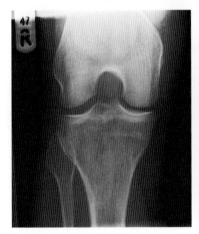

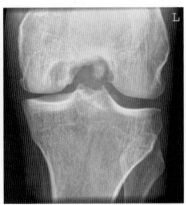

90-degree angulation

110-degree angulation (loose body demonstrated)

KNEE – 'SKYLINE' PATELLA (SUPERO-INFERIOR)

Position of Patient and Image Receptor
- The patient sits on the end or side of the X-ray table, with the knees flexed over the side.
- Ideally, the affected knee should be flexed to 45 degrees.
- Too much flexion reduces the retro-patellar spacing. Sitting the patient on a cushion helps to achieve the optimum position.
- The image receptor is supported horizontally on a stool at the level of the inferior tibial tuberosity border.

Direction and Centring of X-ray Beam
- The vertical beam is directed to the posterior aspect of the proximal border of the patella. The central ray should be parallel to the long axis of the patella.
- The beam is collimated to the patella and femoral condyles.
- Ensure lead protection is given to the patient.

Essential Image Characteristics
- The image should clearly show the patello-femoral joint space.
- Not enough flexion will cause the tibial tuberosity to overshadow the retro-patellar joint.
- Too much flexion will cause the patella to track over the lateral femoral condyle.

Additional Considerations
- There are at least three methods of achieving a skyline patella projection; however, the supero-inferior method is reasonably quick to undertake and has radiation protection advantages.

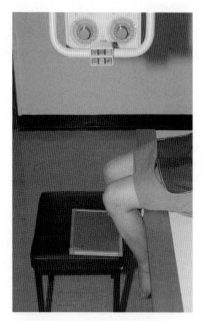

Positioning for skyline patella

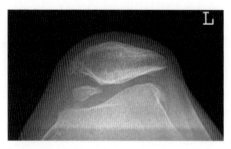

Skyline patella radiograph showing
degenerative changes and loose bone fragment

LUMBAR SPINE – ANTERO-POSTERIOR

Position of Patient and Image Receptor

- The patient lies supine on the Bucky table, with the median sagittal plane coincident with, and at right-angles to, the midline of the table and Bucky.
- The anterior superior iliac spines should be equidistant from the tabletop.
- The hips and knees are flexed and the feet are placed with their plantar aspect on the tabletop to reduce the lumbar arch and bring the lumbar region of the vertebral column parallel with the image receptor.
- The image receptor should be large enough to include the lower thoracic vertebrae and the sacro-iliac joints and is centred at the level of the lower costal margin.
- The exposure should be made on arrested expiration allowing the diaphragm to move superiorly. The air within the lungs would otherwise cause a large difference in density and poor contrast between the upper and lower lumbar vertebrae.

Direction and Centring of X-ray Beam

- Direct the central ray towards the midline at the level of the lower costal margin (L3).

Essential Image Characteristics

- The image should include from T12 down to the bottom of the sacro-iliac joints.
- Rotation can be assessed by ensuring that the sacro-iliac joints are equidistant from the spine.
- The exposure used should produce a density such that bony detail can be discerned throughout the region of interest.

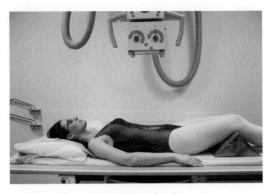

Positioning for antero-posterior lumbar spine

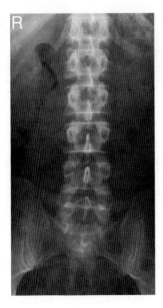

Example of antero-posterior lumbar spine radiograph

LUMBAR SPINE – LATERAL

Position of Patient and Image Receptor

- The patient lies on their side on the Bucky table. If there is any degree of scoliosis, then the most appropriate lateral position will be such that the concavity of the curve is towards the X-ray tube.
- The arms should be raised and resting on the pillow in front of the patient's head. The knees and hips are flexed for stability.
- The coronal plane running through the centre of the spine should coincide with, and be perpendicular to, the midline of the Bucky.
- The image receptor is centred at the level of the lower costal margin.
- The exposure should be made on arrested expiration.
- This projection can also be undertaken erect with the patient standing or sitting.

Direction and Centring of X-ray Beam

- Direct the central ray at right-angles to the line of spinous processes and towards a point 7.5 cm anterior to the third lumbar spinous process at the level of the lower costal margin.

Essential Image Characteristics

- The image should include T12 downwards, to include the lumbar sacral junction.
- Ideally, the projection will produce a clear view through the centre of the intervertebral disc spaces, with individual vertebral endplates superimposed.
- The cortices at the posterior and anterior margins of the vertebral body should also be superimposed.
- The imaging factors selected must produce an image density sufficient for diagnosis from T12 to L5/S1, including the spinous processes.

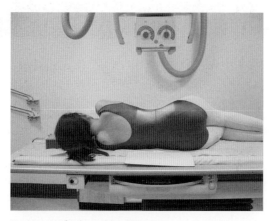

Positioning for lateral lumbar spine

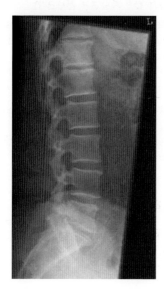

Example of lateral
lumbar spine
radiograph

LUMBAR SPINE – OBLIQUE

Position of Patient and Image Receptor

- The patient is positioned supine on the Bucky table and is then rotated 45 degrees to the right and left sides in turn.
- The hips and knees are flexed and the patient is supported with a 45-degree foam pad placed under the trunk on the raised side.
- The image receptor is centred at the lower costal margin.

Direction and Centring of X-ray Beam

- Direct the vertical central ray towards the midclavicular line on the raised side at the level of the lower costal margin.

Essential Image Characteristics

- The degree of obliquity should be such that the posterior elements of the vertebrae are aligned in such a way as to show the classic 'Scottie dog' appearance.

Notes

- These projections demonstrate the pars interarticularis and the apophyseal joints on the side nearest the image receptor. Both sides are taken for comparison.

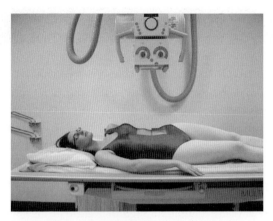

Positioning for right lateral oblique lumbar spine

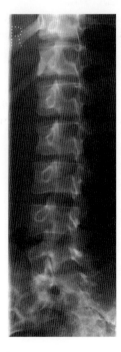

Left posterior
oblique radiograph

LUMBAR SACRAL JUNCTION (L5–S1) – LATERAL

Position of Patient and Image Receptor

- The patient lies on their side on the Bucky table, with the arms raised and the hands resting on the pillow. The knees and hips are flexed slightly for stability.
- The dorsal aspect of the trunk should be at right-angles to the image receptor. This can be assessed by palpating the iliac crests or the posterior superior iliac spines.
- The coronal plane running through the centre of the spine should coincide with, and be perpendicular to, the midline of the Bucky.
- The image receptor is centred at the level of the fifth lumbar spinous process.
- Non-opaque pads may be placed under the waist and knees, as necessary, to bring the vertebral column parallel to the image receptor.

Direction and Centring of X-ray Beam

- Direct the central ray at right-angles to the lumbo-sacral region and towards a point 7.5 cm anterior to the fifth lumbar spinous process. This is found at the level of the tubercle of the iliac crest or midway between the level of the upper border of the iliac crest and the anterior superior iliac spine.
- If the patient has particularly large hips and the spine is not parallel with the tabletop, then a 5-degree caudal angulation may be required to clear the joint space.

Essential Image Characteristics

- The area of interest should include the fifth lumbar vertebra and the first sacral segment.
- A clear joint space should be demonstrated.

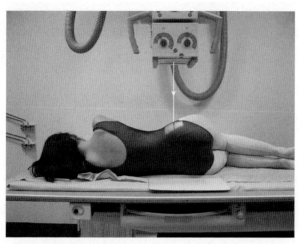

Positioning for lateral L5–S1

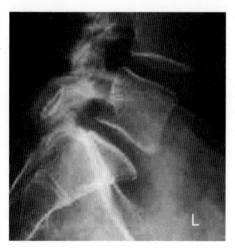

Lumbar sacral junction radiograph

MANDIBLE – POSTERO-ANTERIOR

Position of Patient and Image Receptor

- The projection should be performed erect with the patient seated facing the image receptor (a grid/Bucky should be used).
- The patient's median sagittal plane should be coincident with the midline of the Bucky or image receptor. The head is then adjusted to bring the orbito-meatal baseline perpendicular to the Bucky.
- The median sagittal plane should be perpendicular to the image receptor. Also check that the external auditory meatuses are equidistant from it.
- If an image receptor is used it should be positioned such that its middle, when placed longitudinally in the Bucky or cassette holder, is centred at the level of the angles of the mandible.

Direction and Centring of X-ray Beam

- The central ray is directed perpendicular to the image receptor and centred in the midline at the levels of the angles of the mandible.

Essential Image Characteristics

- The whole of the mandible from the lower portions of the temporo-mandibular joints to the symphysis menti should be included in the image.
- There should be no rotation evident.

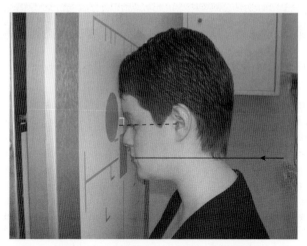

Positioning for postero-anterior mandible projection

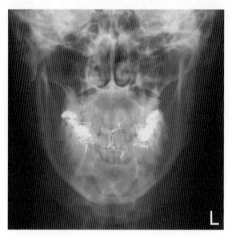

Example of postero-anterior mandible
radiograph

MANDIBLE – LATERAL OBLIQUE

Position of Patient and Image Receptor

- The median sagittal plane should be parallel with the image receptor and the inter-pupillary line perpendicular.
- The neck may be extended slightly to clear the mandible from the spine.
- The image receptor and head can now be adjusted and supported so the above position is maintained but is comfortable for the patient.
- If a CR cassette is used it should be parallel with the long axis of the mandible and the lower border positioned 2 cm below the mandible's lower border.
- The projection may also be performed with a horizontal beam in trauma cases when the patient cannot be moved.
- In this case, the patient will be supine with the median sagittal plane at right-angles to the tabletop. The CR cassette is supported vertically against the side under examination.

Direction and Centring of X-ray Beam

- The central ray is angled 30 degrees cranially at an angle of 60 degrees to the image receptor and is centred 5 cm inferior to the angle of the mandible remote from the image receptor.
- Collimate to include the whole of the mandible and temporo-mandibular joint (include the external auditory meatus within the collimation field).

Essential Image Characteristics

- The body and ramus of each side of the mandible should not be superimposed.
- The image should include the whole of the mandible, from the temporo-mandibular joint to the symphysis menti.

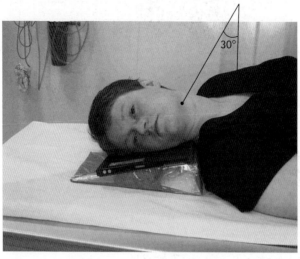

Positioning for lateral oblique mandible projection

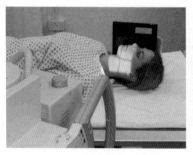

Positioning for trauma lateral oblique mandible projection

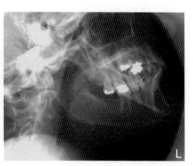

Example of lateral oblique mandible radiograph

ORBITS – OCCIPITO-MENTAL (MODIFIED)

Position of Patient and Image Receptor

- The projection is best performed erect with the patient seated facing the image receptor (a grid/Bucky should be used).
- The head is then adjusted to bring the orbito-meatal baseline to an angle of 35 degrees.
- The horizontal central line of the image receptor should be level with the middle of the orbits and the median sagittal plane should coincide with its vertical central line.
- Ensure that the median sagittal plane is at right-angles to the image receptor by checking the outer canthi of the eyes and the external auditory meatuses are equidistant.

Direction and Centring of X-ray Beam

- The central ray should be perpendicular and central to the image receptor before positioning commences (ensure the X-ray tube and Bucky are at the same height as the patient's head).
- To check that the beam is centred properly, the cross-lines on the Bucky or cassette holder should coincide with the middle line at the level of the orbits.
- Ensure the X-ray tube is recentred to the middle of the image receptor if it is moved during positioning.

Essential Image Characteristics

- The petrous ridges should appear in the lower third maxillary sinuses.
- The orbits should be roughly circular in appearance (they will be more oval in the occipito-mental projection).
- There should be no rotation.

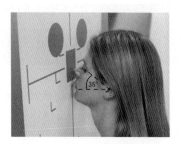

Positioning for orbits projection

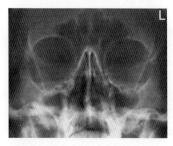

Example of orbits radiograph

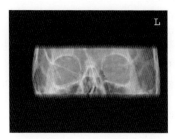

Collimation used for foreign-body
projection

ORTHOPANTOMOGRAPHY (OPG/OPT)

Position of Patient and Image Receptor

- Any bulky clothing and radio-opaque objects, such as jewellery, dentures or hearing aids should be removed from the imaged area.
- The equipment is brought to the start position and careful explanation is given to the patient.
- A 15 × 30 cm image receptor is used on many machines; however, Direct Radiography (DR) technology may be utilized on newer equipment.
- The patient walks into the machine, holding the handles and adopting a 'skiing' position.
- The head is tilted downwards until the Frankfort plane is parallel with the floor and the machine height adjusted to allow the patient to bite into the bite block, with upper and lower incisors within the grooves. The chin should be placed on the rest.
- Ensure the patient is not rotated by ensuring the sagittal plane light runs down the middle of the face. Close the head restraints.
- The patient is asked to place their tongue on the roof of their mouth to reduce the air shadow and is asked to keep still for 20 seconds.
- The exposure is taken. Observe the patent carefully.

Direction and Centring of X-ray Beam

- The antero-posterior light should be centred distally to the upper lateral incisor. This allows optimal positioning of the 'focal trough', the zone of focus outside of which the anatomical detail becomes blurred.

Essential Image Characteristics

- Correct anatomical coverage, which should include the entire mandible and temporo-mandibular joints.
- There should be good contrast and density between the enamel and dentine. The anatomical detail should be clearly defined with optimal resolution if the focal trough has been carefully placed in position.
- Edge-to-edge incisors.
- No removable metallic foreign bodies.
- No evidence of movement unsharpness.
- No evidence of positioning errors, including rotation and errors within the occlusal plane (both external edges of the rami should be parallel to each other).
- The spinal shadow should be minimized.
- The air shadow at the roof of the mouth should be minimized if the tongue was placed correctly.

Additional Considerations

- Problems can occur with producing an optimal image with this technique, due to a number of factors, including patient movement and positioning errors.
- It is essential that the patient is able to co-operate and stay still for up to 20 seconds for a successful examination to take place.

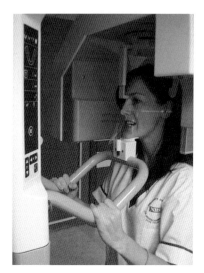

Positioning for OPG

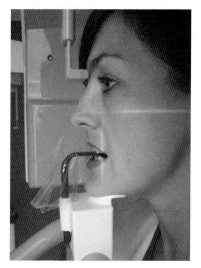

Positioning for OPG

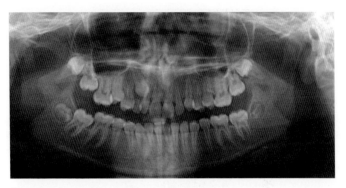

Example of correctly positioned OPG

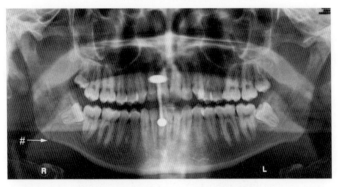

OPG demonstrating a mandibular fracture (#) and 'tongue stud' artefact

PELVIS – ANTERO-POSTERIOR

Position of Patient and Image Receptor

- The patient lies supine with their median sagittal plane perpendicular to the tabletop.
- The midline of the patient must coincide with the centred primary beam and table Bucky mechanism.
- To avoid pelvic rotation, the anterior superior iliac spines must be equidistant from the tabletop.
- The limbs are slightly abducted and internally rotated to bring the femoral necks parallel to the image receptor.

Direction and Centring of X-ray Beam

- Centre in the midline, with a vertical central beam to the centre of the image receptor.
- The centre of the image receptor is placed midway between the upper border of the symphysis pubis and anterior superior iliac spine for the whole of the pelvis and proximal femora. The upper edge of the image receptor should be 5 cm above the upper border of the iliac crest to compensate for the divergent beam and to ensure that the whole of the bony pelvis is included.

Essential Image Characteristics

- Iliac crests and proximal femora, including the lesser trochanters, should be visible on the image.
- No rotation. The iliac bones and obturator foramina should be the same size and shape.

Additional Considerations

- At first visit and trauma cases, gonad protection is usually omitted, however local protocols can vary. It is used on follow-up images.

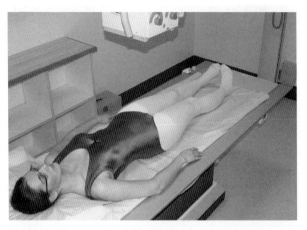

Positioning for antero-posterior pelvis

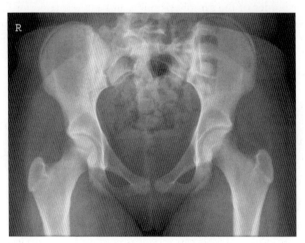

Example of antero-posterior pelvis radiograph

SACRO-ILIAC JOINTS – POSTERO-ANTERIOR

Position of Patient and Image Receptor

- The patient lies prone, with their median sagittal plane perpendicular to the tabletop.
- The posterior superior iliac spines should be equidistant from the tabletop to avoid rotation.
- The midline of the patient should coincide with the centred primary beam and the table Bucky mechanism.
- The forearms are raised and placed on the pillow.
- The image receptor should be displaced inferiorly so that the central ray passes through the centre of the image receptor.

Direction and Centring of X-ray Beam

- Centre in the midline at the level of the posterior superior iliac spines.
- The central ray is angled 5–15 degrees caudally from the vertical, depending on the sex of the patient. The female requires greater caudal angulation of the beam.
- The primary beam is collimated to the area of interest.

Additional Considerations

- The projection may be undertaken in the antero-posterior position but in the postero-anterior position the diverging oblique rays coincide with the direction of the joints, thus demonstrating them more effectively.
- The dose to the gonads and pelvic content is reduced when postero-anterior positioning is employed.

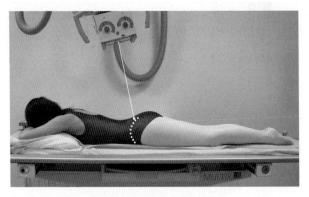

Positioning for postero-anterior sacro-iliac joints

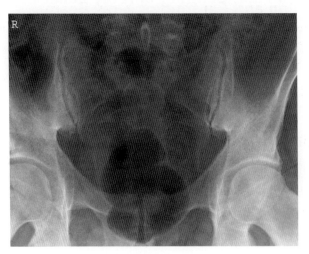

Normal postero-anterior projection of sacro-iliac joints

SACRUM – LATERAL

Position of Patient and Image Receptor

- The patient lies on their side on the Bucky table, with the arms raised and the hands resting on the pillow. The knees and hips are flexed slightly for stability.
- The dorsal aspect of the trunk should be at right-angles to the image receptor. This can be assessed by palpating the iliac crests or the posterior superior iliac spines. The coronal plane running through the centre of the spine should coincide with, and be perpendicular to, the midline of the Bucky.
- The image receptor is centred to coincide with the central ray at the level of the midpoint of the sacrum.

Direction and Centring of X-ray Beam

- Direct the central ray at right-angles to the long axis of the sacrum and towards a point in the midline of the table at a level midway between the posterior superior iliac spines and the sacro-coccygeal junction.

Essential Image Characteristics

- Fractures are easily missed if the exposure is inadequate or a degree of rotation is present.

Additional Considerations

- If using an automatic exposure control, centring too far posteriorly will result in an underexposed image.

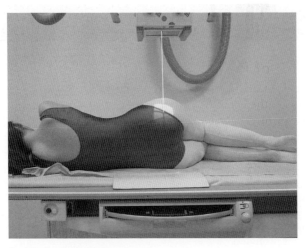

Positioning for lateral sacrum

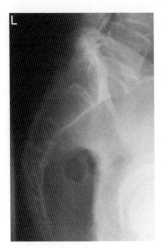

Lateral sacrum radiograph

SCAPHOID – POSTERO-ANTERIOR WITH ULNAR DEVIATION

For suspected scaphoid fractures, three or more projections may be taken: these normally include the postero-anterior and lateral (wrist projections, pp 218–221), plus one or more of the three projections described in this book.

Position of Patient and Image Receptor

- The patient is seated alongside the table with the affected side nearest the table.
- The arm is extended across the table with the elbow flexed and the forearm pronated.
- If possible, the shoulder, elbow and wrist should be at the level of the tabletop.
- The wrist is positioned over the centre of the image receptor and the hand is adducted (ulnar deviation).
- Ensure that the radial and ulnar styloid processes are equidistant from the image receptor.
- The hand and lower forearm are immobilized using sandbags.

Direction and Centring of X-ray Beam

- The vertical central ray is centred midway between the radial and ulnar styloid processes.

Essential Image Characteristics

- The image should include the distal end of the radius and ulna and the proximal end of the metacarpals.
- The joint space around the scaphoid should be demonstrated clearly.

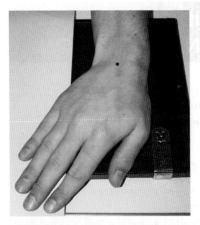

Positioning for postero-anterior
scaphoid with ulnar deviation

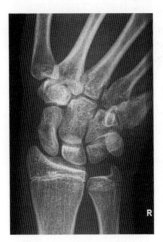

Example of postero-anterior
scaphoid with ulnar deviation

SCAPHOID – ANTERIOR OBLIQUE WITH ULNAR DEVIATION

Position of Patient and Image Receptor
- From the postero-anterior position, the hand and wrist are rotated 45 degrees externally and placed central over an image receptor. The hand should remain adducted in ulnar deviation.
- The hand is supported in position, with a non-opaque pad placed under the thumb.
- The forearm is immobilized using a sandbag.

Direction and Centring of X-ray Beam
- The vertical central ray is centred midway between the radial and ulnar styloid processes.

Essential Image Characteristics
- The image should include the distal end of the radius and ulna and the proximal end of the metacarpals.
- The scaphoid should be seen clearly, with its long axis parallel to the image receptor.

Additional Considerations
- For scaphoid fractures, three or more projections may be taken: these normally include the **postero-anterior and lateral (wrist projections)**, plus one or more of the three projections described in this book.
- A carpal fracture is a break of one of the eight small bones of the carpus. These bones are the scaphoid, lunate, capitate, triquetrum, hamate, pisiform, trapezium and trapezoid. Fractures of the other carpal bones do occur but the scaphoid is accountable for 60–70% of fractures of the carpal bones.

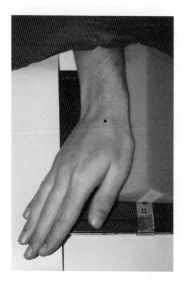

Positioning for anterior oblique scaphoid

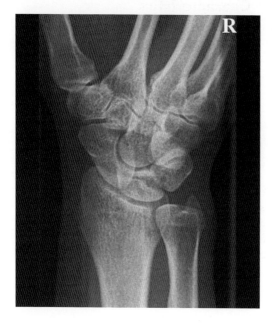

Example radiograph of anterior oblique scaphoid

SCAPHOID – POSTERIOR OBLIQUE

Position of Patient and Image Receptor

- From the anterior oblique position, the hand and wrist are rotated externally through 90 degrees, such that the posterior aspect of the hand and wrist are at 45 degrees to the image receptor.
- The wrist is then supported on a 45-degree non-opaque foam pad.
- The forearm is immobilized using a sandbag.

Direction and Centring of X-ray Beam

- The vertical central ray is centred over the styloid process of the ulna.

Essential Image Characteristics

- The image should include the distal end of the radius and ulna and the proximal end of the metacarpals.
- The pisiform should be seen clearly in profile situated anterior to the triquetral.
- The long axis of the scaphoid should be seen perpendicular to the image receptor.

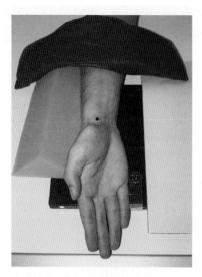

Positioning for posterior oblique
scaphoid

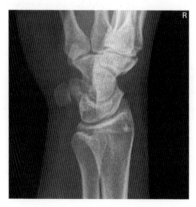

Example of posterior oblique scaphoid
radiograph

SCAPHOID POSTERO-ANTERIOR – ULNAR DEVIATION AND 30-DEGREE CRANIAL ANGLE

The patient and image receptor are positioned as for the postero-anterior scaphoid with ulnar deviation. The wrist must be positioned to allow the X-ray tube to be angled at 30 degrees along the long axis of the scaphoid.

Direction and Centring of X-ray Beam
- The vertical central ray is angled 30 degrees cranially and centred to the scaphoid.

Essential Image Characteristics
- This projection elongates the scaphoid and with ulnar deviation demonstrates the space surrounding the scaphoid.

Notes
- As the X-ray beam is directed towards the patient's trunk radiation protection of the gonads should be applied.

Radiological Considerations
- Fracture of the waist of the scaphoid may not be clearly visible, if at all, at presentation. It carries a high risk of delayed avascular necrosis of the distal pole, which can cause severe disability. If suspected clinically, the patient may be re-examined after 10 days of immobilization, otherwise a technetium bone scan or magnetic resonance imaging (MRI) may offer immediate diagnosis.

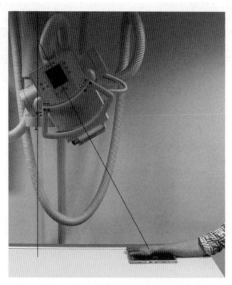

Positioning for a 30-degree angled scaphoid

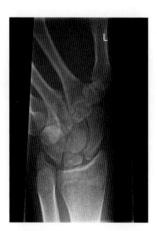

Radiograph of 30-degree
cranial angle

SHOULDER GIRDLE – ANTERO-POSTERIOR

Position of Patient and Image Receptor

- The patient stands with the affected shoulder against the image receptor and is rotated 15 degrees to bring the shoulder closer to the image receptor and the plane of the acromioclavicular joint parallel to the central beam.
- The arm is supinated and slightly abducted away from the body. The medial and lateral epicondyles of the distal humerus should be parallel to the image receptor.
- The image receptor is positioned so that its upper border is at least 5 cm above the shoulder to ensure that the oblique rays do not project the shoulder off the image.

Direction and Centring of X-ray Beam

- The horizontal central ray is directed to the palpable coracoid process of the scapula.
- The central ray passes through the upper glenoid space to separate the articular surface of the humerus from the acromion process.

Essential Image Characteristics

- The image should demonstrate the head and proximal end of the humerus, the inferior angle of the scapula and the whole of the clavicle.
- The head of the humerus should be seen slightly overlapping the glenoid cavity but separate from the acromion process.
- Arrested respiration aids good rib detail in acute trauma.

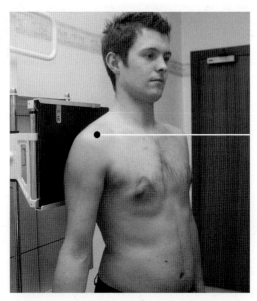

Positioning for antero-posterior shoulder girdle

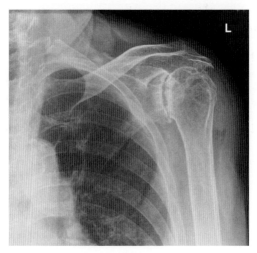

Radiograph of antero-posterior shoulder girdle

SHOULDER JOINT – ANTERO-POSTERIOR (GLENOHUMERAL JOINT)

Position of Patient and Image Receptor

- The patient stands with the affected shoulder against the image receptor and is rotated approximately 30 degrees to bring the plane of the glenoid fossa perpendicular to the image receptor.
- The arm is supinated and slightly abducted away from the body.
- The image receptor is positioned so that its upper border is at least 5 cm above the shoulder to ensure that the oblique rays do not project the shoulder off the cassette.

Direction and Centring of X-ray Beam

- The horizontal central ray is centred to the palpable coracoid process of the scapula.
- The primary beam is collimated to include the head, the greater and lesser tuberosities of the humerus, together with the lateral aspect of the scapula and the distal end of the clavicle.

Essential Image Characteristics

- The image should demonstrate clearly the joint space between the head of the humerus and the glenoid cavity.

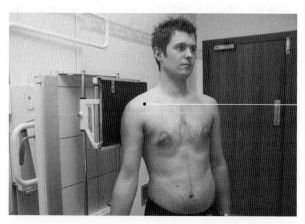

Positioning for antero-posterior shoulder joint projection

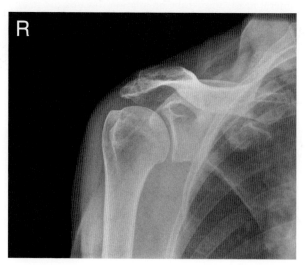

Radiograph of antero-posterior shoulder joint

SHOULDER – SUPERO-INFERIOR (AXIAL)

Position of Patient and Image Receptor

- The patient is seated at the side of the table, which is lowered to waist level.
- The arm under examination is abducted over the image receptor.
- The patient leans forward to reduce the object-to-detector distance and to ensure that the glenoid cavity is included in the image.
- The elbow can remain flexed, but the arm should be abducted to a minimum of 45 degrees, injury permitting.

Direction and Centring of X-ray Beam

- The vertical central ray is directed through the proximal aspect of the humeral head. Some tube angulation towards the palm of the hand may be necessary to coincide with the plane of the glenoid cavity.
- If there is a large object-to-detector distance, it may be necessary to increase the overall focus receptor distance to reduce magnification.

Essential Image Characteristics

- The image should demonstrate the head of the humerus, the acromion process, the coracoid process and the glenoid cavity of the scapula.

Notes

- The most common type of dislocation of the shoulder is an anterior dislocation, where the head of the humerus displaces below the coracoid process, anterior to the glenoid cavity.

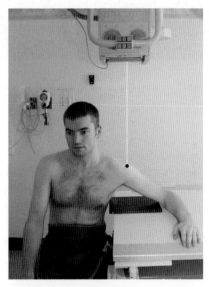

Positioning for axial shoulder

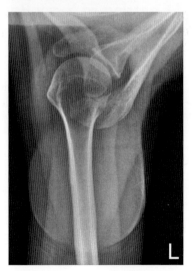

Radiograph for axial shoulder

SHOULDER JOINT – LATERAL OBLIQUE 'Y' PROJECTION

If the arm is immobilized and no abduction of the arm is possible, then a lateral oblique 'Y' projection is taken.

Position of Patient and Image Receptor

- The patient stands or sits with the lateral aspect of the injured arm against the image receptor and is adjusted so that the axilla is in the centre.
- The unaffected shoulder is raised to make the angle between the trunk and image receptor approximately 60 degrees. A line joining the medial and lateral borders of the scapula is now at right-angles to the image receptor.
- The image receptor is positioned to include the superior border of the scapula.

Direction and Centring of X-ray Beam

- The horizontal central ray is directed towards the medial border of the scapula and centred to the head of the humerus.

Essential Image Characteristics

- The body of the scapula should be at right-angles to the image receptor with the scapula and the proximal end of the humerus clear of the rib cage.
- The exposure should demonstrate the position of the head of the humerus in relation to the glenoid cavity between the coracoid and acromion processes.

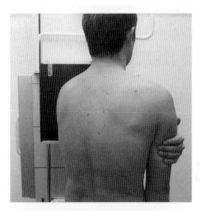

Positioning for lateral oblique 'Y'
projection

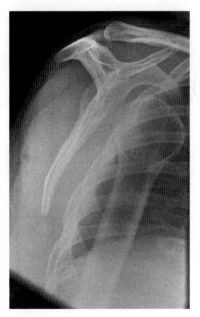

Radiograph lateral oblique 'Y'
projection showing anterior dislocation

SINUSES – OCCIPITO-MENTAL

Position of Patient and Image Receptor

- The projection should be performed erect with the patient seated facing the image receptor (a grid/Bucky should be used).
- The head is then adjusted to bring the orbito-meatal baseline to an angle of 45 degrees to the horizontal.
- The horizontal central line of the image receptor should be level with the lower orbital margins and the median sagittal plane should coincide with its vertical central line.
- Ensure that the median sagittal plane is at right-angles to the image receptor by checking the outer canthi of the eyes and the external auditory meatuses are equidistant from the image receptor.
- The patient should open their mouth wide before the exposure. This will allow demonstration of the sphenoid sinuses through the mouth.

Direction and Centring of X-ray Beam

- The central ray should be perpendicular and central to the image receptor before positioning commences (ensure the X-ray tube and Bucky are at the same height as the patient's head).
- To check that the beam is centred properly, the cross-lines on the Bucky or cassette holder should coincide with the patient's anterior nasal spine.
- Ensure the X-ray tube is re-centred to the middle of the image receptor if it is moved during positioning.
- Collimate to include all of the sinuses.

Essential Image Characteristics

- The petrous ridges must appear below the floors of the maxillary sinuses.
- There should be no rotation.

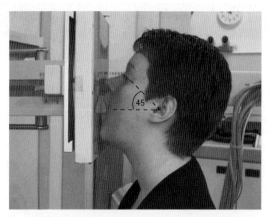

Positioning for occipito-mental sinuses projection

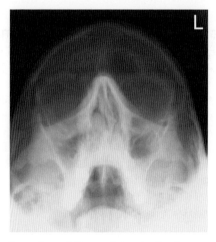

Example occipito-mental projection for
sinuses showing a polyp in right
maxillary sinus

181

SINUSES – OCCIPITO-FRONTAL 15 DEGREES

Position of Patient and Image Receptor

- The projection should be performed erect with the patient seated facing the image receptor (a grid/Bucky should be used).
- The head is positioned so that the orbito-meatal baseline is raised 15 degrees to the horizontal.
- Ensure that the nasion is positioned in the centre of the Bucky.
- The patient may place the palms of the hands either side of the head (out of the primary beam) for stability.

Direction and Centring of X-ray Beam

- The central ray is directed perpendicular to the vertical Bucky along the median sagittal plane so the beam exits at the nasion.
- A collimation field should be set to include the ethmoidal and frontal sinuses. The size of the frontal sinuses can vary drastically from one individual to another.

Essential Image Characteristics

- All the frontal and ethmoid sinuses should be visualized within the image.
- The petrous ridges should be projected just above the lower orbital margin.
- It is important to ensure that the skull is not rotated. This can be assessed by measuring the distance from a point in the midline of the skull to the lateral orbital margins. If this is the same on both sides of the skull, then it is not rotated.

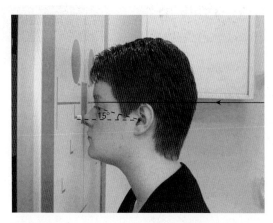

Positioning for occipito-frontal 15-degree sinuses projection

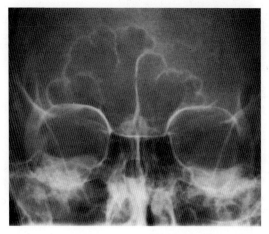

Example of occipito-frontal 15-degree projection for sinuses

SINUSES – LATERAL

Position of Patient and Image Receptor

- The patient sits facing the vertical Bucky. The head is then rotated, such that the median sagittal plane is parallel to the Bucky and the inter-orbital line is perpendicular to the Bucky.
- The shoulders may be rotated slightly to allow the correct position to be attained. The patient may grip the Bucky for stability.
- The head and Bucky heights are adjusted so that the centre of the Bucky is 2.5 cm along the orbito-meatal line from the outer canthus of the eye.
- A radiolucent pad may be placed under the chin for support.

Direction and Centring of X-ray Beam

- A horizontal central ray should be employed to demonstrate fluid levels.
- The X-ray tube should have been centred previously to the Bucky, such that the central ray will now be centred to a point 2.5 cm posterior to the outer canthus of the eye.

Essential Image Characteristics

- A true lateral will have been achieved if the lateral portions of the floors of the anterior cranial fossa are superimposed.

Additional Considerations

- This projection may also be undertaken with the patient supine and the cassette supported vertically against the side of the face. Again, a horizontal beam is used to demonstrate fluid levels.

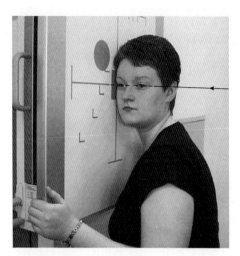

Positioning for lateral sinuses projection

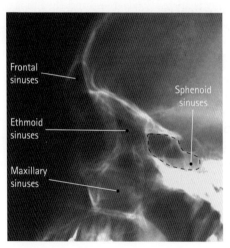

Frontal
sinuses

Sphenoid
sinuses

Ethmoid
sinuses

Maxillary
sinuses

Example of lateral sinuses radiograph

SKULL – OCCIPITO-FRONTAL 20 DEGREES↓

Position of Patient and Image Receptor

- This projection may be undertaken erect or in the prone position (erect positioning described).
- The patient is seated facing the erect Bucky, so that the median sagittal plane is coincident with the midline of the Bucky and is also perpendicular to it.
- The neck is flexed so that the orbito-meatal baseline is perpendicular to the Bucky. This can usually be achieved by ensuring that the nose and forehead are in contact with the Bucky.
- Ensure that the mid-part of the frontal bone is positioned in the centre of the Bucky.

Direction and Centring of X-ray Beam

- The central ray is angled 20 degrees caudally and is aligned to the median sagittal plane.
- A collimation field should be set to include the vertex of the skull superiorly, the region immediately below the base of the occipital bone inferiorly, and the lateral skin margins. It is important to ensure that the tube is centred to the middle of the Bucky.

Essential Image Characteristics

- All the cranial bones should be included within the image, including the skin margins.
- It is important to ensure that the skull is not rotated.
- The petrous ridges should appear just below the inferior orbital margin.

Additional Considerations

- The same result can be achieved by raising the orbito-meatal baseline by 20 degrees with no caudal angulation applied to the tube (see image).

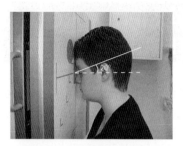

Positioning for occipito-frontal (OF) 20°↓ skull projection

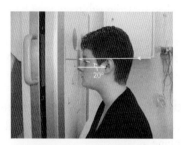

Alternative positioning for occipito-frontal (OF) 20°↓ skull using straight tube with the orbito-meatal baseline raised 20°

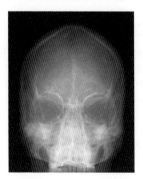

Example of occipito-frontal (OF) 20°↓ radiograph

187

SKULL – OCCIPITO-FRONTAL 30 DEGREES↑ (REVERSE TOWNE'S)

Position of Patient and Image Receptor

- This projection is usually undertaken with the patient in the erect position and facing the erect Bucky, although it may be performed prone.
- Initially, the patient is asked to place their nose and forehead on the Bucky table. The head is adjusted to bring the median sagittal plane at right-angles to the image receptor and so it is coincident with its midline.
- The orbito-meatal baseline should be perpendicular to the image receptor.
- The patient may place their hands on the Bucky for stability.

Direction and Centring of X-ray Beam

- The central ray is angled cranially so it makes an angle of 30 degrees to the orbito-meatal plane.
- Adjust the collimation field, such that the whole of the occipital bone and the parietal bones up to the vertex are included within the field. Avoid including the eyes in the primary beam. Laterally, the skin margins should also be included within the field.

Essential Image Characteristics

- The sella turcica of the sphenoid bone is projected within the foramen magnum.
- The image must include all of the occipital bone and the posterior parts of the parietal bone, and the lambdoidal suture should be visualized clearly.
- The skull should not be rotated. This can also be assessed by ensuring that the sella turcica appears in the middle of the foramen magnum.

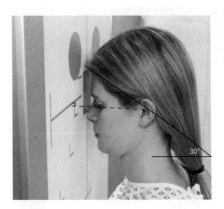

Positioning for reverse Towne's projection

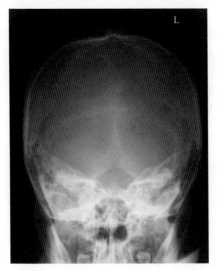

Example of 30 degree↑ radiograph

SKULL – LATERAL ERECT

Position of Patient and Image Receptor

- The patient sits facing the erect Bucky and the head is then rotated, such that the median sagittal plane is parallel to the Bucky and the inter-orbital line is perpendicular to it.
- The shoulders may be rotated slightly to allow the correct position to be attained. The patient may grip the Bucky for stability.
- Position the image receptor transversely in the erect Bucky, such that its upper border is 5 cm above the vertex of the skull.
- A radiolucent pad may be placed under the chin for support.

Direction and Centring of X-ray Beam

- The X-ray tube should have been centred previously to the Bucky.
- Adjust the height of the Bucky/tube so that the patient is comfortable. (NB: do not decentre the tube from the Bucky at this point.)
- Centre midway between the glabella and the external occipital protuberance to a point approximately 5 cm superior to the external auditory meatus.

Essential Image Characteristics

- The image should contain all of the cranial bones and the first cervical vertebra. Both the inner and outer skull tables should be included.
- A true lateral will result in perfect superimposition of the lateral portions of the floors of the anterior cranial fossa and those of the posterior cranial fossa.

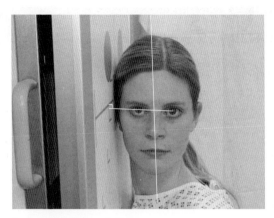

Positioning for lateral skull

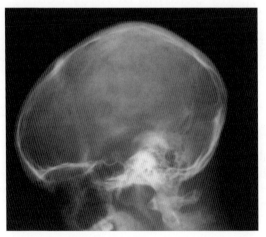

Lateral skull radiograph

SKULL – FRONTO-OCCIPITAL 20 DEGREES↑ (SUPINE/TROLLEY)

Position of Patient and Image Receptor

- The patient lies supine on a trolley or Bucky table, or with the posterior aspect of the skull resting against the image receptor (a grid should be employed).
- The head is adjusted to bring the median sagittal plane at right-angles to the image receptor and coincident with its midline. In this position, the external auditory meatuses are equidistant from the image receptor.
- The orbito-meatal baseline should be perpendicular to the image receptor.

Direction and Centring of X-ray Beam

- The central ray is angled 20 degrees cranially and directed to the image receptor or Bucky along the median sagittal plane.
- A collimation field should be set to include the vertex of the skull superiorly, the base of the occipital bone inferiorly, and the lateral skin margins. It is important to ensure that the X-ray tube is centred to the middle of the image receptor/Bucky.

Essential Image Characteristics

- See occipito-frontal projection page 186.

Additional Considerations

- Alternative technique: in the example given opposite an fronto-occipital (FO)20°↑ projection is required, but the patient can only maintain their orbito-meatal baseline in a position 10 degrees back from perpendicular (i.e. with the chin raised slightly). In order to achieve an overall 20-degree angle, a 10-degree cranial angulation will need to be applied to the tube.

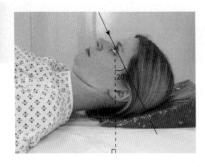

Positioning for FO20°↑

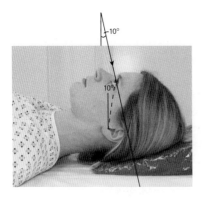

FO20°↑ projection achieved with
10-degree tube angle and RBL raised
10 degrees

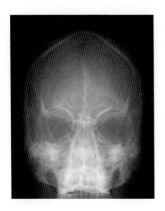

Example of FO20°↑ radiograph

SKULL – MODIFIED HALF AXIAL[1] (SUPINE/TROLLEY)

Position of Patient and Image Receptor

- The patient lies supine on a trolley or Bucky table, with the posterior aspect of the skull resting on the image receptor (a grid should be employed).
- The head is adjusted to bring the median sagittal plane at right-angles to the image receptor so it is coincident with its midline.
- The orbito-meatal baseline should be perpendicular to the image receptor.

Direction and Centring of X-ray Beam

- The central ray is angled caudally so it makes an angle of 25 degrees to the orbito-meatal plane.
- Set a collimation field such that its lower border is limited immediately above the supra-orbital ridges at their highest point. The upper border of the light beam should just include the vertex of the skull at its highest point. Collimate laterally to include the skin margins within the field.
- The top of the CR cassette (if used) should be positioned adjacent to the vertex of the skull to ensure that the beam angulation does not project the area of interest off the bottom of the image.

Essential Image Characteristics

- The sella turcica of the sphenoid bone is projected within the foramen magnum.
- The image must include all of the occipital bone and the posterior parts of the parietal bone, and the lambdoidal suture should be visualized clearly.
- The skull should not be rotated. This can also be assessed by ensuring that the sella turcica appears in the middle of the foramen magnum.

[1]Denton BK (1998) Improving plain radiography of the skull: the half axial projection re-described. *Synergy* August: 9–11.

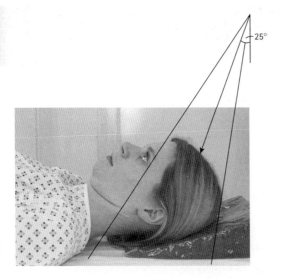

25°

Positioning for
modified half axial

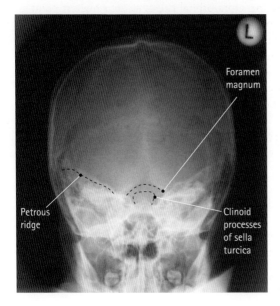

L

Foramen
magnum

Petrous
ridge

Clinoid
processes
of sella
turcica

Example of modified
half axial radiograph

SKULL – LATERAL (SUPINE/TROLLEY)

Position of Patient and Image Receptor

- The patient lies supine, with the head raised and immobilized on a non-opaque skull pad. This will ensure that the occipital region is included on the final image.
- The head is adjusted, such that the median sagittal plane is perpendicular to the table/trolley and the inter-orbital line is perpendicular to the image receptor.
- Support the image receptor with grid vertically against the lateral aspect of the head parallel to the median sagittal plane, with its long edge 5 cm above the vertex of the skull.

Direction and Centring of X-ray Beam

- The horizontal central ray is directed parallel to the inter-orbital line, such that it is at right-angles to the median sagittal plane.
- Centre midway between the glabella and the external occipital protuberance to a point approximately 5 cm superior to the external auditory meatus.
- The long axis of the cassette should be coincident with the long axis of the skull.

Essential Image Characteristics

- The image should contain all of the cranial bones and the first cervical vertebra. Both the inner and outer skull tables should be included.
- A true lateral will result in perfect superimposition of the lateral portions of the floors of the anterior cranial fossa and those of the posterior cranial fossa.

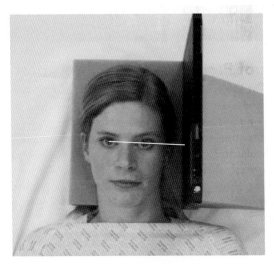

Positioning for lateral supine skull (anterior aspect)

MSP

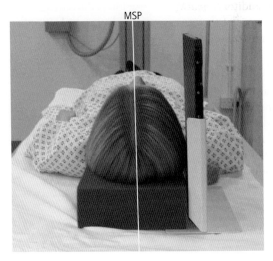

Positioning for lateral supine skull (superior aspect)

STERNUM – LATERAL

Position of Patient and Image Receptor

- The patient sits or stands, with either shoulder against a vertical Bucky or image receptor stand.
- The patient's feet are separated for stability.
- The median sagittal plane of the trunk is adjusted parallel to the image receptor.
- The sternum is centred to the image receptor.
- The patient's hands are clasped behind the back and the shoulders are pulled well back immediately before the exposure on arrested inspiration.
- The image receptor is centred at a level 2.5 cm below the sternal angle.

Direction and Centring of X-ray Beam

- Direct the horizontal central ray towards a point 2.5 cm below the sternal angle.
- An FRD of 150 cm should be used to reduce magnification.

Essential Image Characteristics

- This can be a difficult examination to interpret, especially in elderly patients, who often have heavily calcified costal cartilages.
- The image should demonstrate the full extent of the sternum, including the manubrium, body and xiphoid process.
- The contrast and density should be optimized to demonstrate the cortical margins of the sternum.

Additional Considerations

This projection is usually taken in conjunction with a chest radiograph to search for a pneumothorax in trauma cases.

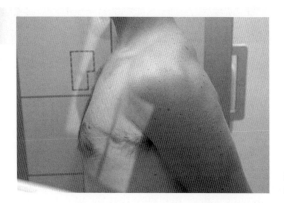

Positioning for lateral sternum

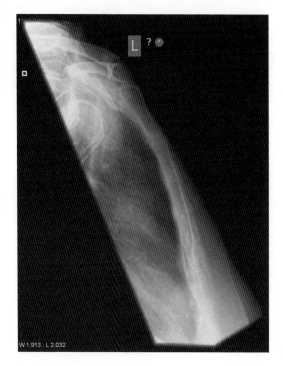

Example of lateral sternum radiograph

THORACIC SPINE – ANTERO-POSTERIOR

Position of Patient and Image Receptor

- The patient is positioned supine on the X-ray table, with the median sagittal plane perpendicular to the tabletop and coincident with the midline of the Bucky.
- The upper edge of an image receptor, which should be at least 40 cm long for an adult, should be at a level just below the prominence of the thyroid cartilage to ensure that the upper thoracic vertebrae are included.
- Make exposure on arrested inspiration. This will cause the diaphragm to move down over the upper lumbar vertebrae, thus reducing the chance of a large density difference appearing on the image from superimposition of the lungs.

Direction and Centring of X-ray Beam

- Direct the central ray at right-angles to the image receptor and towards a point 2.5 cm below the sternal angle.
- Collimate tightly to the spine.

Essential Image Characteristics

- The image should include vertebrae from C7 to L1.
- The image density should be sufficient to demonstrate bony detail for the upper as well as the thoracic lower vertebrae.

Additional Considerations

- The image receptor and beam are often centred too low, thereby excluding the upper thoracic vertebrae from the image.
- The lower vertebrae are also often not included. L1 can be identified easily by the fact that it usually will not have a rib attached to it.

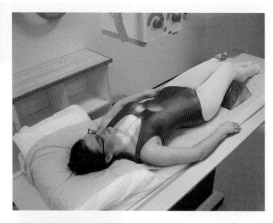

Positioning for
antero-posterior
thoracic spine

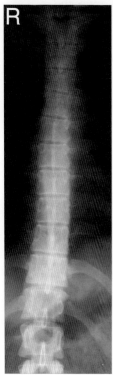

Example of antero-posterior
thoracic spine image

THORACIC SPINE – LATERAL

Position of Patient and Image Receptor

- Usually undertaken with the patient in the lateral decubitus position on the X-ray table.
- The median sagittal plane should be parallel to the image receptor and the midline of the axilla coincident with the midline of the table or Bucky.
- The arms should be raised well above the head.
- The head can be supported with a pillow, and pads may be placed between the knees for the patient's comfort.
- The upper edge of the image receptor should be 3–4 cm above the spinous process of C7. The image receptor should be at least 40 cm long.

Direction and Centring of X-ray Beam

- The central ray should be at right-angles to the long axis of the thoracic vertebrae. This may require a caudal angulation.
- Centre 5 cm anterior to the spinous process of T6–T7. This is usually found just below the inferior angle of the scapula (assuming the arms are raised), which is easily palpable.

Essential Image Characteristics

- The upper two or three vertebrae may not be demonstrated due to the superimposition of the shoulders.
- Look for the absence of a rib on L1 at the lower border of the image. This will ensure that T12 has been included within the field.
- The posterior ribs should be superimposed, thus indicating that the patient was not rotated too far forwards or backwards.

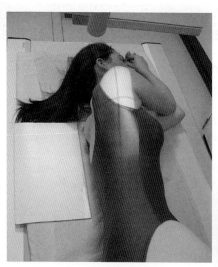

Positioning for lateral thoracic spine

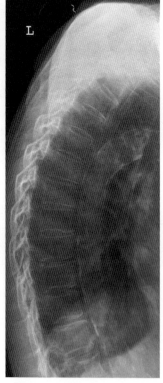

Example of lateral thoracic spine radiograph

THUMB – ANTERO-POSTERIOR

Position of Patient and Image Receptor

- The patient is seated facing away from the table with the arm extended backwards and medially rotated at the shoulder. The hand may be slightly rotated to ensure that the second, third and fourth metacarpals are not superimposed on the base of the first metacarpal.
- The patient leans forward, lowering the shoulder so that the first metacarpal is parallel to the tabletop.
- The image receptor is placed under the wrist and thumb and oriented to the long axis of the metacarpal.

Direction and Centring of X-ray Beam

- The vertical central ray is centred over the first metacarpo-phalangeal joint.

Essential Image Characteristics

- Where there is a possibility of injury to the base of the first metacarpal, the carpo-metacarpal joint must be included on the image.

Additional Considerations

- The image should include the fingertip and the distal third of the metacarpal bone.

Notes

- The postero-anterior projection increases object-to-film distance and hence, potentially, unsharpness, but it is sometimes easier and less painful for the patient.
- The use of the postero-anterior projection maintains the relationship of the adjacent bones, i.e. the radius and ulna, which is essential in cases of suspected foreign body in the thenar eminence.

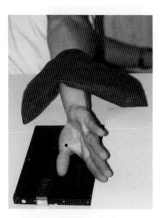

Positioning for antero-posterior thumb

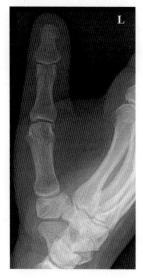

Example of antero-posterior thumb radiograph

THUMB – LATERAL

Position of Patient and Image Receptor

- The patient is seated alongside the table with the arm abducted, the elbow flexed and the anterior aspect of the forearm resting on the table.
- The thumb is flexed slightly and the palm of the hand is placed on the image receptor.
- The palm of the hand is raised slightly with the fingers partially flexed and supported on a non-opaque pad, such that the lateral aspect of the thumb is in contact with the image receptor.

Direction and Centring of X-ray Beam

- The vertical central ray is centred over the first metacarpo-phalangeal joint.

Essential Image Characteristics

- Where there is a possibility of injury to the base of the first metacarpal, the carpo-metacarpal joint must be included on the image.
- The image should include the fingertip and the distal third of the metacarpal bone.

Notes

- It is common practice to obtain two projections, a lateral and an antero-posterior. In the case of a suspected foreign body in the thenar eminence, a postero-anterior projection is used to maintain the relationship with adjacent structures.

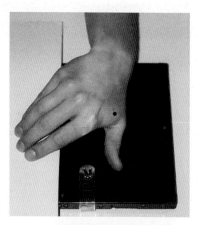

Positioning for lateral thumb

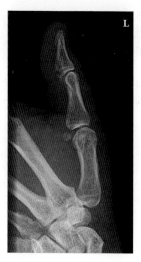

Example of lateral thumb
radiograph

TIBIA AND FIBULA – ANTERO-POSTERIOR

Position of Patient and Image Receptor

- For CR, a 35 × 43-cm image receptor is used for adults, with the lower leg placed diagonally to ensure the full length of the tibia and fibula is included.
- The patient is either supine or seated on the X-ray table, with both legs extended.
- The ankle is supported in dorsi-flexion by a firm 90-degree pad placed against the plantar aspect of the foot. The limb is rotated medially until the medial and lateral malleoli are equidistant from the image receptor.
- The lower edge of the image receptor is positioned just below the plantar aspect of the heel.

Direction and Centring of X-ray Beam

- Centre to the middle of the image receptor, with the central ray at right-angles to both the long axis of the tibia and an imaginary line joining the malleoli.

Essential Image Characteristics

- The knee and ankle joints should be included on the image. This is especially important in trauma, as a break in the bony ring may be accompanied by another fracture within the ring (such as the distal tibia and proximal fibula).

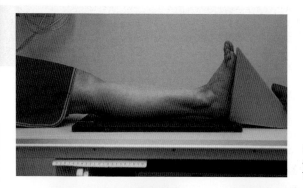

Positioning for
antero-posterior
tibia and fibula

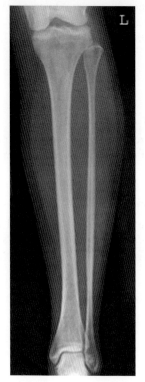

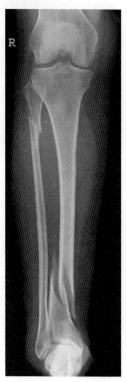

Examples of antero-posterior tibia and fibula radiographs. The
right image demonstrates proximal fibula and distal tibial fractures

TIBIA AND FIBULA – LATERAL

Position of Patient and Image Receptor

- From the supine/seated position, the patient rotates onto the affected side.
- The leg is rotated further until the malleoli are superimposed vertically.
- The tibia should be parallel to the image receptor.
- A pad is placed under the knee for support.
- The lower edge of the image receptor is positioned just below the plantar aspect of the heel.

Direction and Centring of X-ray Beam

- Centre to the middle of the image receptor, with the central ray at right-angles to the long axis of the tibia and parallel to an imaginary line joining the malleoli.

Essential Image Characteristics

- The knee and ankle joints should be included on the image.

Additional Considerations

- If it is impossible to include both joints on one image, then two images should be exposed separately, one to include the ankle and the other to include the knee. Both images should include the middle third of the lower leg, so the general alignment of the bones may be seen.
- If the patient cannot turn into the lateral position, an adapted technique utilizing a horizontal beam and image receptor resting against the medial aspect of the lower leg is used.

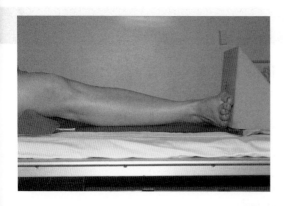

Positioning for lateral tibia and fibula

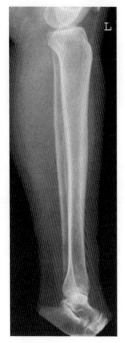

Tibia and fibula (normal)

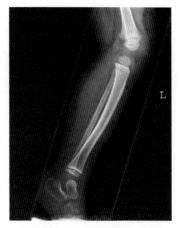

Tibia and fibula (fractured)

TOE – HALLUX – LATERAL

Position of Patient and Image Receptor

- From the dorsi-plantar position, the foot is rotated medially until the medial aspect of the hallux is in contact with the image receptor.
- A bandage is placed around the remaining toes (provided that no injury is suspected) and they are gently pulled forwards by the patient to clear the hallux.
- Alternatively, they may be pulled backwards; this shows the metatarso-phalangeal joint more clearly.

Direction and Centring of X-ray Beam

- The vertical ray is centred over the first metatarso-phalangeal joint.

Essential Image Characteristics

- The image should demonstrate the phalanges and shaft of the first metatarsal.
- The remaining toes should be pulled clear of the phalanges with minimal overlapping.

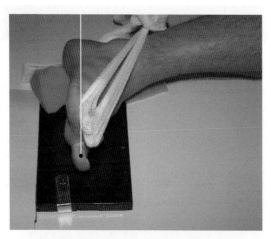

Positioning for lateral hallux

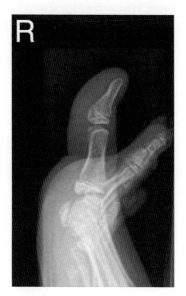

Example of lateral hallux
radiograph

TOES – DORSI-PLANTAR

Position of Patient and Image Receptor

- The patient is seated on the X-ray table, supported if necessary, with hips and knees flexed.
- The plantar aspect of the affected foot is placed on the image receptor. This image receptor may be supported on a 15-degree pad.
- The leg may be supported in the vertical position by the other knee.

Direction and Centring of X-ray Beam

- The vertical central ray is directed over the third metatarso-phalangeal joint, perpendicular to the image receptor if all the toes are to be imaged.
- For single toes, the vertical ray is centred over the metatarso-phalangeal joint of the individual toe and collimated to include the toe either side.

Essential Image Characteristics

- The image should demonstrate the full area of interest, including the distal phalanges and proximal metatarsal region.
- A uniform radiographic contrast across the area of interest is desirable.

Additional Considerations

- It is common practice to obtain two projections, a dorsi-plantar and dorsi-plantar oblique.
- True lateral projections of the toes are generally not requested, except in the case of the big toe, where a dorsi-plantar and lateral are the accepted standard.

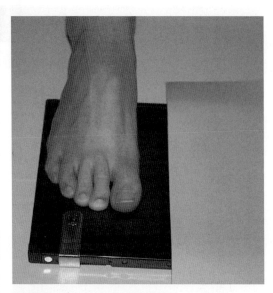

Positioning for dorsi-plantar toes

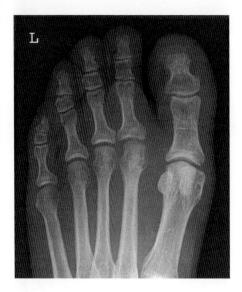

Example of dorsi-plantar toes
radiograph

215

TOES SECOND TO FIFTH – DORSI-PLANTAR OBLIQUE

Position of Patient and Image Receptor

- From the basic dorsi-plantar position, the affected limb is allowed to lean medially to bring the plantar surface of the foot approximately 45 degrees to the image receptor.
- A 45-degree non-opaque pad is placed under the side of the foot for support, with the opposite leg acting as a support.

Direction and Centring of X-ray Beam

- The vertical ray is centred over the first metatarso-phalangeal joint if all the toes are to be imaged and angled sufficiently to allow the central ray to pass through the third metatarso-phalangeal joint.
- For single toes, the vertical ray is centred over the metatarso-phalangeal joint of the individual toe, perpendicular to the image receptor.

Essential Image Characteristics

- The image should demonstrate the full area of interest, including the distal phalanges and proximal metatarsal region.
- A uniform radiographic contrast across the area of interest is desirable.

Additional Considerations

- Ensure foot is not over-rotated medially, which may result in toes overlapping each other.

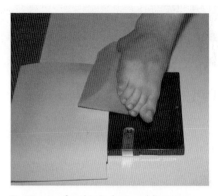

Positioning for dorsi-plantar oblique toes

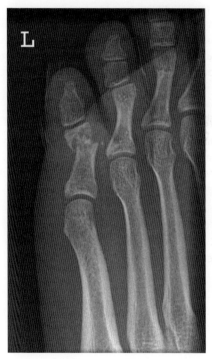

Fractured fifth proximal phalanx

WRIST – POSTERO-ANTERIOR

Position of Patient and Image Receptor

- The patient is seated alongside the table, with the affected side nearest to the table.
- The elbow joint is flexed to 90 degrees and the arm is abducted, such that the anterior aspect of the forearm and the palm of the hand rests on the image receptor.
- If the mobility of the patient permits, the shoulder joint should be at the same height as the forearm.
- The wrist joint is placed central to the image receptor and adjusted to include the lower part of the radius and ulna and the proximal two-thirds of the metacarpals.
- The fingers are flexed slightly to bring the anterior aspect of the wrist into contact with the image receptor.
- The wrist joint is adjusted to ensure that the radial and ulnar styloid processes are equidistant from the image receptor.
- The forearm is immobilized using a sandbag.

Direction and Centring of X-ray Beam

- The vertical central ray is centred to a point midway between the radial and ulnar styloid processes.

Essential Image Characteristics

- The image should demonstrate the proximal two-thirds of the metacarpals, the carpal bones, and the distal third of the radius and ulna.
- There should be no rotation of the wrist joint.

Notes

- When the image is undertaken for a scaphoid view the wrist should be in ulnar deviation.

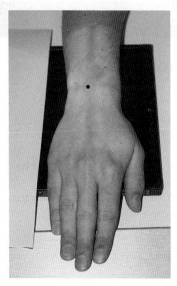

Positioning for postero-anterior
wrist

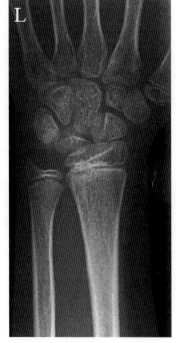

Radiograph of postero-anterior
wrist

WRIST – LATERAL

Position of Patient and Image Receptor

- The patient is seated alongside the table, with the affected side nearest to the table.
- The elbow joint is extended to bring the medial aspect of the forearm, wrist and hand into contact with the table.
- The wrist joint is positioned to include the lower part of the radius and ulna and the proximal two-thirds of the metacarpals on the image receptor.
- The hand is rotated externally slightly further to ensure that the radial and styloid processes are superimposed.
- The forearm is immobilized using a sandbag.

Direction and Centring of X-ray Beam

- The vertical central ray is centred over the styloid process of the radius.

Essential Image Characteristics

- The image should demonstrate the proximal two-thirds of the metacarpals, the carpal bones, and the distal third of the radius and ulna.
- There should be no rotation of the wrist joint.

Notes

- If the elbow is extended rather than at right-angles it is often easier to rotate the wrist into a lateral position.

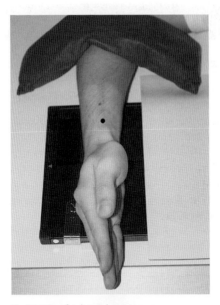

Positioning for lateral wrist

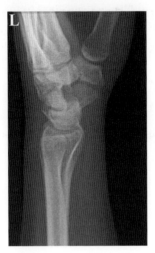

Example of lateral wrist
radiograph

ZYGOMATIC ARCHES – INFERO-SUPERIOR

Position of Patient and Image Receptor

- The patient lies supine, with one or two pillows under the shoulders to allow the neck to be extended fully.
- The image receptor is placed against the vertex of the skull, such that its long axis is parallel with the axial plane of the body. It should be supported in this position with foam pads and sandbags.
- The flexion of the neck is now adjusted to bring the long axis of the zygomatic arch parallel to the image receptor.
- The head is now tilted 5–10 degrees away from the side under examination. This allows the zygomatic arch under examination to be projected onto the image receptor without superimposition of the skull vault or facial bones.

Direction and Centring of X-ray Beam

- The central ray should be perpendicular to the image receptor and long axis of the zygomatic arch.
- A centring point should be located such that the central ray passes through the space between the midpoint of the zygomatic arch and the lateral border of the facial bones.
- Tight collimation can be applied to reduce scatter and to avoid irradiating the eyes.

Essential Image Characteristics

- The whole length of the zygomatic arch should be demonstrated clear of the skull.

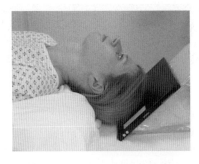

Positioning for
zygomatic arches

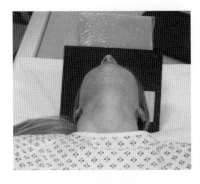

Positioning for
zygomatic arches

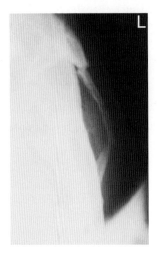

Zygomatic arch radiograph
demonstrating double
fracture

SECTION 3

USEFUL INFORMATION FOR RADIOGRAPHIC PRACTICE

NON-IMAGING DIAGNOSTIC TESTS

The following blood tests are commonly performed as part of the diagnostic process. The results may have an impact upon the appropriateness of certain imaging procedures or raise suspicions of particular pathology. The reader should consult local departmental protocols for guidance in relation to some of these tests and their significance.

D-dimer

A test that measures the levels of products from the degradation of fibrin within blood clots. Raised D-dimer levels increase the suspicion of conditions such a pulmonary embolism and deep vein thrombosis. Low D-dimer levels can be used to exclude the possibility of these conditions and the need to perform expensive imaging tests.

INR: International Normalized Ratio

A measure of the time taken for blood to clot. A normal result would be around 1 but patients who are taking anticoagulant drugs may have a value of 2.0–3.5. Invasive diagnostic tests, such as angiography, may be contraindicated with patients with a high INR due to the subsequent risk of haemorrhage (see local departmental protocols for guidance).

e-GFR: Estimated Glomerular Filtration Rate

Used to measure the health of the kidneys and renal function. It takes into account variables such as age, gender and serum creatinine levels. Levels of greater than $90\,mL/minute/1.73\,m^2$ are considered normal. Levels below this value indicate impaired renal function.

ESR: Erythrocyte Sedimentation Rate

A non-specific test which measures the time taken for red blood cells to settle in a thin tube of liquid. Various diseases will affect the ability of the cells to do this and will increase the time taken for the cells to settle. Some examples of such diseases include those which cause inflammation, autoimmune diseases, cancers or myeloma. Typical normal values for adults are between 10–20 mm/hour. This value varies considerably with age. Values of over 100 would be of significant concern.

SCr: Serum Creatinine

Creatinine is a metabolic waste product that is excreted from the blood plasma by the kidneys. A raised serum creatinine indicates impaired renal function (normal levels are typically in the range 0.6–1.2 mg/dL). Patients with raised serum creatinine may be at an increased risk from renal failure if iodinated contrast agents are administered (see local departmental protocols for guidance).

LFTs: Liver Function Tests

A group of tests that is used to assess the overall health of the liver and biliary system. Abnormal tests can give early indications of serious conditions. If the liver is diseased and the cells are damaged, various enzymes will be released into the blood stream, e.g. alanine transaminase (ALT) or alkaline phosphatase (ALP). Disease may also affect the ability of the liver to produce albumin. High levels of bilirubin in the blood indicate jaundice.

MEDICAL TERMINOLOGY

The following list of common prefixes and suffixes can be employed to work out the meaning of complex disease terminology encountered on requests for radiological examinations.

Prefixes

A– or An–	absence of or without
Adreno–	relating to the adrenal glands
Angio–	relating to blood or lymph vessels
Ante–	in front or before
Arterio–	relating to arteries
Brady–	slow
Bucc–	relating to the cheek
Burs–	relating to bursa within synovial joints
Cardi–	relating to the heart
Cephal–	relating to the head
Cervi–	relating to the neck
Cerebr–	relating to the brain
Chol–	relating to the biliary system or bile
Crani–	relating to the skull
Cysto–	relating to the bladder or gall bladder
Dacro–	relation to tears and associated glands or ducts
Dys	difficulty
Ec–	away from or not in usual position
Endo–	inside or within
Ente–	relating to the intestine
Epi–	upon
Ex–	out of
Gastr–	relating to the stomach
Gingiv–	relating to the gums
Haem–	relating to the blood
Hemi–	half
Hydro–	water
Hyper–	beyond normal limits

Hypo–	below normal limits
Hystro–	relating to the uterus
Idio–	relating to an individual or self
Infra–	below
Inter–	between
Iso–	the same as
Lact–	milk
Laparo–	relating to the abdomen wall
Leuco–	relating to white blood cells
Lingu–	relating to the tongue
Lipo–	fat
Litho–	stone formation
Lympho–	relating to the lymphatic system
Lysis–	destruction of
Macro–	large
Mammo or masto–	relating to the breast
Mega–	enlargement of
Myo–	muscle
Neo–	new
Nephro–	relating to kidney
Neuro–	relating to the nervous system
Osteo–	relating to the bones
Orchid–	relating to the testes
Peri–	around
Phleb–	relating to the veins
Pneumo–	relating to the lungs
Poly–	many
Post–	after
Pyo–	pus
Retro–	behind
Salpingo–	relating to the uterine tubes
Sial–	relating to the salivary glands
Spleno–	relating to the spleen
Spondy–	relating to the spine
Sub–	beneath
Tachy–	too fast
Trach–	relating to the trachea

Trans–	through
Urin– or uro–	relating to the urinary system or urine
Vesico–	relating to the bladder

Suffixes

–aemia	disease affecting the blood
–algia	pain
–ectasis	enlargement of
–ectomy	the surgical removal of
–itis	inflammation of
–oma	tumour
–oscopy	the visual examination of
–ostomy	surgical opening of
–osis	disease of
–penia	lack of
–plasty	repair or reconstruction
–rrhoea	flow

MEDICAL ABBREVIATIONS

AAA	abdominal aortic aneurysm
ACL	anterior cruciate ligament
AE	air entry
AF	atrial fibrillation
AFP	alpha-fetoprotein
ALL	acute lymphocytic leukaemia
AML	acute myelogenous leukaemia
AP	antero-posterior
ARDS	acute respiratory distress syndrome
ASD	atrial septal defect
AVM	arteriovenous malformation
AXR	abdomen X-ray
BaE or BE	barium enema
BI	bony injury
BMI	body mass index
BP	blood pressure
Ca	cancer
CT	computed tomography
CAT	computed axial tomography
CABG	coronary artery bypass graft
CBD	common bile duct
COPD	chronic obstructive pulmonary disease
CO	complains of
CN	cranial nerve
CPR	cardiopulmonary resuscitation
CR	computed radiography
CTR	cardiothoracic ratio
CSF	cerebrospinal fluid
CVA	cerebrovascular accident (stroke)
CVP	central venous pressure
CXR	chest X-ray

D&V	diarrhoea and vomiting
D&C	dilation and curettage
DVT	deep vein thrombosis
DIP	distal interphalangeal (joint)
DDx	differential diagnosis
DNA	did not attend
DX	diagnosis
DXT	deep X-ray treatment
ECG	electrocardiogram
ECT	electroconvulsive therapy
EDD	estimated date of delivery
ENT	ear, nose and throat
ESR	erythrocyte sedimentation rate
ET	endotracheal
ERCP	endoscopic retrograde cholangio-pancreatography
FBC	full blood count
FB	foreign body
FH	family history
FO	fronto-occipital
FTT	failure to thrive
FUO	fever of unknown origin
GCS	Glasgow coma scale
GIT	gasterointestinal tract
GFR	glomerular filtration rate
GU	gastric ulcer or genito-urinary
Hb	haemoglobin
HI	head injury
HIV	human immunodeficiency virus
Hx	history of
IAM	internal auditory meatus
IDDM	insulin-dependent diabetes mellitus

IDK	internal derangement of the knee
IM	intramedullary or intramuscular
IVC	inferior vena cava or intravenous cholangiogram
IVP	intravenous pyelogram
IVU	intravenous urogram
KUB	kidneys, ureters and bladder
LAO	left anterior oblique
LLL	left lower lobe
LMP	last menstrual period
LOC	loss of consciousness
LP	lumbar puncture
LUL	left upper lobe
LUQ	left upper quadrant
LVF	left ventricular failure
MCP	metacarpo-phalangeal
MI	myocardial infarction
MRI	magnetic resonance imaging
MRSA	methicillin resistant *Staphylococcus aureus*
MS	multiple sclerosis or mitral stenosis
MSP	median sagittal plane
NAD	no abnormality detected
NBI	no bony injury
NBM	nil by mouth
NFR	not for resuscitation
NFS	no fracture seen
NG	nasogastric or new growth
NIDDM	non-insulin dependent diabetes mellitus
NMR	nuclear magnetic resonance
NSAIDs	non-steroidal anti-inflammatory drugs
NSCLC	non small cell lung caranoma
OA	osteoarthritis
OE	on examination

OF	occipito-frontal
OM	occipito-mental
ORIF	open reduction and internal fixation
PA	postero-anterior
PE	pulmonary embolus
PID	prolapsed intervertebral disc or pelvic inflammatory disease
PIJ	proximal interphalangeal joint
PNS	post-nasal space
POP	plaster of Paris
PR	per (via) the rectum
PRN	as often as needed
PTCA	percutaneous transluminal coronary angioplasty
PUO	pyrexia of unknown origin
PV	per (via) the vagina
RA	rheumatoid arthritis
RAO	right anterior oblique
RBC	red blood cell
RLL	right lower lobe
RML	right middle lobe
ROI	region of interest
RT	radiotherapy
RTC	road traffic collision
RUL	right upper lobe
RUQ	right upper quadrant
Rx	treatment
SAH	subarachnoid haemorrhage
SBE	subacute bacterial endocarditis
SLE	systemic lupus erythematosus
SMV	submentovertical
SOL	space occupying lesion
SOB	shortness of breath
SXR	skull X-ray
STD	sexually transmitted disease
Sx	symptoms

TB	tuberculosis
TFT	thyroid function test
THR	total hip replacement
TIA	transient ischaemic attack
TKR	total knee replacement
TMJ	temporo-mandibular joint
TPR	temperature, pulse and respiration
TURP	transurethral resection of prostate
Tx	treatment

UC	ulcerative colitis
US	ultrasound
URTI	upper respiratory tract infection
UTI	urinary tract infection
U&E	urea and electrolytes

VF	ventricular fibrillation
V/Q	lung perfusion/ventilation scan
VSD	ventricular septal defect
VT	ventricular tachycardia

| WBC | white blood cell count |

| YO | years old |

0	not present
+	present
++	present significantly
+++	present substantially
↑/↓	increase/decrease
#	fracture
1/7	1 day
2/52	2 weeks
3/12	3 months

INDEX

Note: page numbers in **bold** refer to figures/information contained in tables.